AF342303

Mathematics and Visualization

Series Editors

Gerald Farin
Hans-Christian Hege
David Hoffman
Christopher R. Johnson
Konrad Polthier

Springer

Berlin
Heidelberg
New York
Barcelona
Hong Kong
London
Milan
Paris
Tokyo

Ravikanth Malladi

Editor

Geometric Methods in Bio-Medical Image Processing

With 70 Figures, 18 in Color

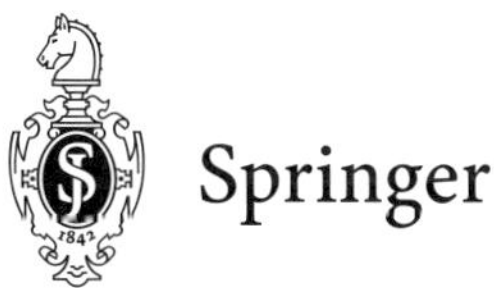

Springer

Editor

Ravikanth Malladi

50A-1148 Lawrence Berkeley National Laboratory
University of California at Berkeley
1, Cyclotron Rd.
Berkeley, CA 94720, USA
e-mail: malladi@euphrates.lbl.gov

Cataloging-in-Publication Data applied for

Die Deutsche Bibliothek - CIP-Einheitsaufnahme

Geometric methods in bio-medical image processing /
Ravikanth Malladi ed.. -
Berlin ; Heidelberg ; New York ; Barcelona ; Hong Kong ;
London ; Milan ; Paris ; Tokyo : Springer, 2002
(Mathematics and visualization)
ISBN 3-540-43216-7

Mathematics Subject Classification (2000): 92C55, 94A08

ISBN 3-540-43216-7 Springer-Verlag Berlin Heidelberg New York

Springer-Verlag Berlin Heidelberg New York
a member of BertelsmannSpringer Science+Business Media GmbH

http://www.springer.de

© Springer-Verlag Berlin Heidelberg 2002
Printed in Germany

Typeset by the authors using a Springer TeX macro package
Cover design: *design & production* GmbH, Heidelberg

SPIN 10846830   46/3142LK - 5 4 3 2 1 0 – Printed on acid-free paper

Preface

It gives me great pleasure to edit this book. The genesis of this book goes back to the conference held at the University of Bologna in June 1999, on collaborative work between the University of California at Berkeley and the University of Bologna. The original idea was to invite some speakers at the conference to submit articles to the book. The scope of the book was later enhanced and, in the present form, it is a compilation of some of the recent work using geometric partial differential equations and the level set methodology in medical and biomedical image analysis.

The synopsis of the book is as follows: In the first chapter, R. Malladi and J. A. Sethian point to the origins of the use of level set methods and geometric PDEs for segmentation, and present fast methods for shape segmentation in both medical and biomedical image applications. In Chapter 2, C. Ortiz de Solorzano, R. Malladi, and S. J. Lockett describe a body of work that was done over the past couple of years at the Lawrence Berkeley National Laboratory on applications of level set methods in the study and understanding of confocal microscope imagery. The work in Chapter 3 by A. Sarti, C. Lamberti, and R. Malladi addresses the problem of understanding difficult time varying echocardiographic imagery. This work presents various level set models that are designed to fit a variety of imaging situations, i.e. time varying $2D$, $3D$, and time varying $3D$. In Chapter 4, L. Vese and T. F. Chan present a segmentation model without edges and also show extensions to the Mumford-Shah model. This model is particularly powerful in certain applications when comparisons between normal and abnormal subjects is required. Next, in Chapter 5, A. Elad and R. Kimmel use the fast marching method on triangulated domain to build a technique to unfold the cortex and map it onto a sphere. This technique is motivated in part by new advances in fMRI based neuroimaging. In Chapter 6, T. Deschamps and L. D. Cohen present a minimal path based method of grouping connected components and show clever applications in vessel detection in $3D$ medical data. Finally, in Chapter 7, A. Sarti, K. Mikula, F. Sgallari, and C. Lamberti, describe a nonlinear model for filtering time varying $3D$ medical data and show impressive results in both ultrasound and echo images.

I owe a debt of gratitude to Claudio Lamberti and Alessandro Sarti for inviting me to Bologna, and logistical support for the conference. I thank the contributing authors for their enthusiasm and flexibility, the Springer mathematics editor Martin Peters for his optimism and patience, and J. A. Sethian for his unfailing support, good humor, and guidance through the years.

Berkeley, California
October, 2001R. Malladi

Contents

1 Fast Methods for Shape Extraction in Medical and Biomedical Imaging *

R. Malladi and J. A. Sethian

Lawrence Berkeley National Laboratory
and
Department of Mathematics, University of California at Berkeley,
50A-1148, 1 Cyclotron Road, Berkeley, CA 94720, U.S.A.
E-mail: malladi@euphrates.lbl.gov, sethian@math.berkeley.edu

Abstract. We present a fast shape recovery technique in $2D$ and $3D$ with specific applications in modeling shapes from medical and biomedical imagery. This approach and the algorithms described is similar in spirit to our previous work in [16,18], is topologically adaptable, and runs in $O(N \log N)$ time where N is the total number of points visited in the domain. Our technique is based on the level set shape recovery scheme introduced in [16,3] and the fast marching method in [27] for computing solutions to static Hamilton–Jacobi equations.

1.1 Introduction

In many medical applications such as cardiac boundary detection and tracking, tumor volume quantification etc., accurately extracting shapes in $2D$ and $3D$ from medical images becomes an important task. These shapes are implicitly present in noisy images and the idea is to construct their boundary descriptions. Visualization and further processing like volume computation is then possible. Although many techniques exist for the aforementioned, computational time has often been a concern. In this paper, we present a shape modeling technique with specific applications in medical and biomedical image analysis that retains all the advantages and sophistication of existing techniques and executes in real-time.

Active contour [9] and surface models [33] have been used by many researchers to segment objects from medical image data. These models are based on deforming a trial shape towards the boundary of the desired object. The deformation is achieved via solving Euler-Lagrange equations which attempt to minimize an energy functional. As an alternative, implicit surface evolution models have been introduced by Malladi *et al.* [16,18] and Caselles *et al.* [3]. In these models, the curve and surface models evolve under an implicit speed law containing two terms, one that attracts it to the object boundary and the other that is closely related to the regularity of the shape.

* Supported in part by the Applied Mathematical Sciences Subprogram of the Office of Energy Research, U.S. Dept. of Energy under Contract DE-AC03-76SD00098 and by the NSF ARPA under grant DMS-8919074.

One of the challenges in shape recovery is to account for changes in topology as the shapes evolve. In the Lagrangian perspective, this can be done by reparameterizing the curve once every few time steps and to monitor the merge/split of various curves based on some criteria; see [21]. However, some problems still remain in $3D$ where the issue of monitoring topological transformations calls for an elegant solution. In [17,18], the authors have modeled anatomical shapes as propagating fronts moving under a curvature dependent speed function [26]. They adopted the level set formulation of interface motion due to Osher and Sethian [22]. The central idea here is to represent a curve as the zero level set of a higher dimensional function; the motion of the curve is then embedded within the motion of the higher dimensional surface. As shown in [22], this approach offers several advantages. First, although the higher dimensional function remains a function, its zero level set can change topology, and form sharp corners. Second, a discrete grid can be used together with finite differences to devise a numerical scheme to approximate the solution. Third, intrinsic geometric quantities like normal and curvature of the curve can be easily extracted from the higher dimensional function. Finally, everything extends directly to moving surfaces in three dimensions.

In order to isolate shapes from images, an artificial speed term has been synthesized and applied to the front which causes it to stop near object boundaries; see [17,18] for details. In [4,10], this work has been improved by adding an additional term to the governing equation. That work views the object detection problem as computation of curves of minimal (weighted) distance. The extra term is a projection of an attractive force vector on the curve normal. Subsequently the level set based schemes for shape recovery have been extended to $3D$ in [12,5] and geometric measurements from detected anatomical shapes were made in [19]. Finally, interested readers are referred to [10,31,35,15,19] for closely related efforts.

One drawback of the level set methodology stems from computational expense. By embedding a curve as the zero-level set of a higher dimensional function, we have turned a two-dimensional problem into a three-dimensional one. Reducing the added computational expense without sacrificing the other advantages of level set schemes has been the focus of some recent work. Tube or narrow-band methods both in $2D$ and $3D$ have been developed and used in [6,18,1,12]. The main idea of the tube method is to modify the level set method so that it only affects points close to the region of interest, namely the cells where the front is located. Another way to reduce the complexity of level set method is adaptive mesh refinement. This is precisely what Milne [20] has done in his thesis. The basic idea here is to start with a relatively coarse grid and adaptively refine the grid based on proximity to the zero level set or at places with high curvature. In both these cases it is possible to reduce computational expense from $O(M^3)$ to $O(M^2)$ per time step in the case of a moving surface, where M is the number of points in each coordinate direction.

Multi-scale implementation has also been considered as a possibility for fast solution of the level set equation [35].

In this paper, we solve the shape modeling problem by using the fast marching methods devised by Sethian [27,28] and extended to a wider class of Hamilton-Jacobi equations in [2]. The marching method is a numerical technique for solving the Eikonal equation, and results from combining upwind schemes for viscosity solutions of Hamilton-Jacobi equations, narrowband level set methods, and a *min*-heap data structure. It results in a time complexity of $O(N \log N)$, where N is the total number of points in the domain. Some early applications of this algorithm include photolithography in [29], a comparison of this approach with volume-of-fluid techniques in [8], and a fast algorithm for image segmentation in [11], see also [34] for a different Dijkstra-like algorithm which obtains the viscosity solution through a control-theoretic discretization which hinges on a causality relationship based on the optimality criterion. We note that an abbreviated version of this work was first reported in Malladi and Sethian [11]. A lot of related efforts have been reported in the literature since then; we refer the reader to some of them in [23,24,7].

The rest of this paper is organized as follows: section 1.2 introduces the fast marching method; section 1.3 explains shape recovery with the marching method and how it ties together with the level set method [18,12]; section 1.4 presents some results in $2D$ and $3D$.

1.2   The Fast Marching Method

We now briefly discuss the fast marching algorithm introduced in [27], which we shall need for shape recovery. Let Γ be the initial position of a hypersurface and let F be its speed in the normal direction. In the level set perspective, one views Γ as the zero level set of a higher dimensional function $\psi(x, y, z)$. Then, by chain rule, an evolution equation for the moving hypersurface can be produced [22], namely

$$\psi_t + F(x, y, z) \mid \nabla \psi \mid = 0, \tag{1.1}$$

Consider the special case of a monotonically advancing surface, i.e. a surface moving with speed $F(x, y, z)$ that is always positive (or negative). Now, let $T(x, y, z)$ be the time at which the surface crosses a given point (x, y, z). The function $T(x, y, z)$ then satisfies the equation

$$\mid \nabla T \mid F = 1; \tag{1.2}$$

this simply says that the gradient of arrival time is inversely proportional to the speed of the surface. Broadly speaking, there are two ways of approximating the position of the moving surface; iteration towards the solution by numerically approximating the derivatives in Eqn. 1.1 on a fixed Cartesian grid, or explicit construction of the solution function $T(x, y, z)$ from Eqn. 1.2. Our marching algorithm relies on the latter approach.

For the following discussion, we limit ourselves to a two-dimensional problem. Using the correct "entropy" satisfying [26,22] approximation to the gradient, we are therefore looking for a solution in the domain to the following equation:

$$[\max(D_{i,j}^{-x}T, 0)^2 + \min(D_{i,j}^{+x}T, 0)^2 \\ + \max(D_{i,j}^{-y}T, 0)^2 + \min(D_{i,j}^{+y}T, 0)^2]^{1/2} = 1/F_{i,j}, \tag{1.3}$$

where D^- and D^+ are backward and forward difference operators. Since the above equation is in essence a quadratic equation for the value at each grid point, we can iterate until convergence by solving the equation at each grid point and selecting the largest possible value as the solution. This is in accordance with obtaining the correct viscosity solution.

1.2.1   The algorithm

The key to constructing the fast algorithm is the observation that the upwind difference structure of Eqn. 1.3 means that information propagates from smaller values of T to larger values. Hence, the algorithm rests on building a solution to Eqn. 1.3 outwards from the smallest T value. Motivated by the methods in [1,18], the "building zone" is confined to a narrow band around the front. The idea is to sweep the front ahead in an upwind fashion by considering a set of points in the narrow band around the current front, and to march this narrow band forward. We explain this algorithmically:

To illustrate, imagine that one wants to solve the Eikonal equation on an M by M grid on the unit box $[0, 1] \times [0, 1]$ with right-hand-side $F_{i,j} > 0$; furthermore, we are given an initial set $T = 0$ along the top of the box.

1. Initialize
   (a) (Alive Points): Let *Alive* be the set of all grid points at which the value of T is fixed. In our example, $Alive = \{(i, j) : i \in \{1, .., M\}, j = M\}$.
   (b) (Narrow Band Points): Let *NarrowBand* be the set of all grid points in the narrow band. For our example $NarrowBand = \{(i, j) : i \in \{1, .., M\}, j = M - 1\}$, also set $T_{i,M-1} = dy/F_{ij}$, where dy is the spatial step size along y axis.
   (c) (Far Away Points): Let *FarAway* be the set of all the rest of the grid points $\{(i, j) : j < M - 1\}$, set $T_{i,j} = \infty$ for all points in *FarAway*.
2. Marching Forwards
   (a) Begin Loop: Let $(i_{\min}, j_{\min})$ be the point in *NarrowBand* with the smallest value for T.
   (b) Add the point $(i_{\min}, j_{\min})$ to *Alive*; remove it from *NarrowBand*.

(c) Tag as neighbors any points $(i_{\min}-1, j_{\min})$, $(i_{\min}+1, j_{\min})$, $(i_{\min}, j_{\min}-1)$, $(i_{\min}, j_{\min}+1)$ that are not *Alive*; if the neighbor is in *FarAway*, remove it from that set and add it to the *NarrowBand* set.

(d) Recompute the values of T at all neighbors according to Equation (1.3), solving the quadratic equation given by our scheme.

(e) Return to top of Loop.

For more general initial conditions, and for a proof that the above algorithm produces a viable solution, see [2,30].

1.2.2 The Min-Heap data structure

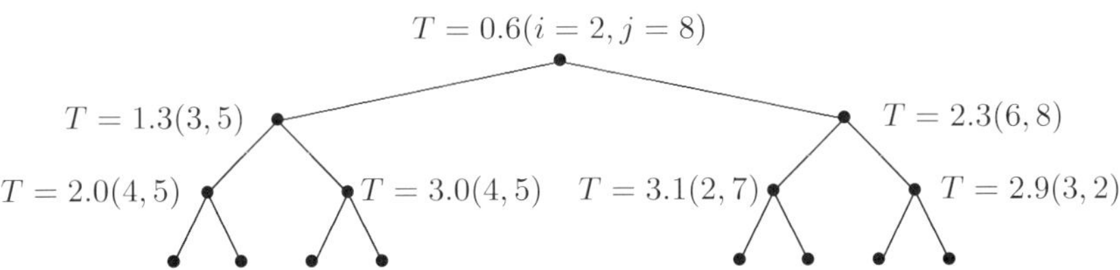

Step 1: Change T value at (2,7)

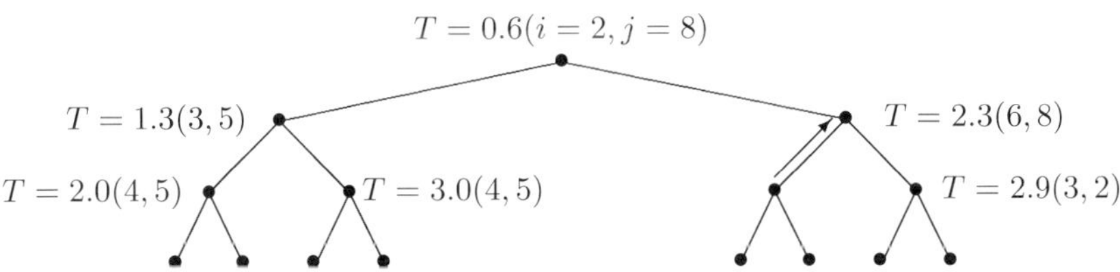

Step 2: New value at (2,7); **UpHeap**

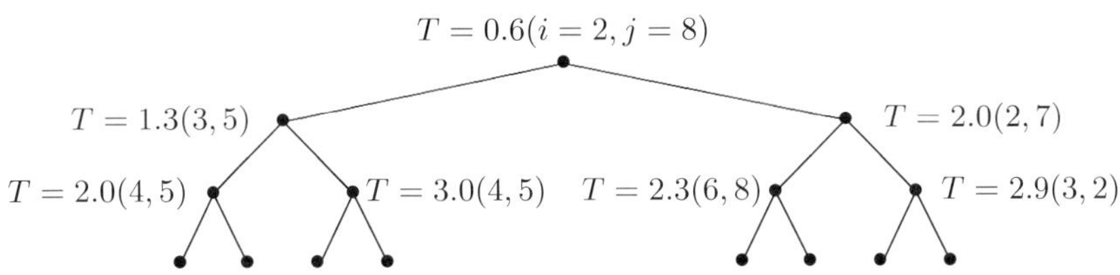

Heap property restored

Fig. 1.1. Heap structure and the **UpHeap** operation

An efficient version of the above technique relies on a fast way of locating the grid point in the narrow band with the smallest value for T. We use a variation on a heap algorithm (see Segdewick [25]) with back pointers to store the T values.

Specifically, we use a min-heap data structure. In an abstract sense, a min-heap is a "complete binary tree" with a property that the value at any given node is less than or equal to the values at its children. In practice, it is more efficient to represent a heap sequentially as an array by storing a node at location k and its children at locations $2k$ and $2k+1$. From this definition, the parent of a given node at k is located at $\lfloor \frac{k}{2} \rfloor$. Therefore, the root which contains the smallest element is stored at location $k = 1$ in the array. Finding the parent or children of a given element are simple array accesses which take $O(1)$ time.

We store the values of T together with the indices which give their location in the grid structure. Our marching algorithm works by first looking for the smallest element in the $NarrowBand$; this `FindSmallest` operation involves deleting the root and one sweep of `DownHeap` to ensure that the remaining elements satisfy the heap property. The algorithm proceeds by tagging the neighboring points that are not $Alive$. The $FarAway$ neighbors are added to the heap using an `Insert` operation and values at the remaining points are updated using Equation 1.3. `Insert` works by increasing the heap size by one and trickling the new element upward to its correct location using an `UpHeap` operation. Lastly, to ensure that the updated T values do not violate the heap property, we need to perform a `UpHeap` operation starting at that location and proceeding up the tree.

The `DownHeap` and `UpHeap` operations (in the worst case) carry an element all the way from root to bottom or vice versa. Therefore, this takes $O(\log M)$ time assuming there are M elements in the heap. It is important to note that the heap which is a complete binary tree is always guaranteed to remain balanced. This leaves us with the operation of searching for the $NarrowBand$ neighbors of the smallest element in the heap. We make this $O(1)$ in time by maintaining back pointers from the grid to the heap array. Without the back pointers, the above search takes $O(M)$ in the worst case. The example in Fig. 1.1 shows the heap structure as the value at location $(2, 7)$ changes from 3.1 to 2.0.

1.3   Shape Recovery from Medical Images

Given a noisy image function $I(\mathbf{x})$, $\mathbf{x} \in \mathcal{R}^2$ for a 2D image and $\mathbf{x} \in \mathcal{R}^3$ in $3D$, the objective in shape modeling is to extract mathematical descriptions of certain anatomical shapes contained in it. We are interested in recovering boundary representation of these shapes with minimal user interaction. In general, our approach consists of starting from user-defined "seed points" in the image domain and to grow trial shape models from these points. These surfaces are made to propagate in the normal direction with a speed $F(\mathbf{x})$.

Shape recovery is possible if we synthesize a special image-based speed function which is defined as a decreasing function of image gradient $|\nabla I(\mathbf{x})|$. The image-based speed function, say k_I, controls the outward propagation of an initial surface (an interior point or a set of interior points) such that the shape model stops in the vicinity of shape boundaries. Mathematically this procedure corresponds to solving a static Hamilton-Jacobi equation (see Eqn. 1.1) which, when recast in the arrival time framework, is

$$| \nabla T(\mathbf{x}) |= \frac{1}{k_I}.\tag{1.4}$$

The speed function defined as

$$F(\mathbf{x}) = k_I(\mathbf{x}) = e^{-\alpha|\nabla G_\sigma * I(\mathbf{x})|}, \ \ \alpha > 0,\tag{1.5}$$

has values very close to zero near high image gradients, i.e., possible edges. False gradients due to noise can be avoided by applying a Gaussian smoothing filter or more sophisticated edge-preserving smoothing schemes (see [13–15,12,32]).

As an example, we consider the problem of reconstructing the entire cortical structure of the human brain from a dense MRI data set. The data is given as intensity values on a $256 \times 256 \times 124$ grid. We start by defining "seed" points in the domain. The value of T at these points is set to zero and the initial heap is constructed from their neighbors. The fast marching algorithm in $3D$ is then employed to march ahead to fill the grid with time values according to Eqn. 1.2. We visualize various stages of our reconstruction by rendering particular level surfaces of the final time function $T(x, y, z)$. These stages are shown in Fig. 1.2. The corrugated structure shown in Fig. 1.2, the level surface $\{T(x, y, z) = 0.75\}$, is our final shape. In Fig. 1.4, we slice the surface parallel to the xy plane and superimpose the resulting contours on the corresponding image. The timings for various stages of calculation on a Sun SPARC 1000 machine are shown in Fig. 1.3. This time is well under 10 seconds on recent SunBlade 1000 machines.

With this model, the surface does not always stop near the shape boundary unless the speed values are very close to zero. More often than not, there are variations in the gradient along the object boundary which can cause the shape to "over-shoot". In large part, the definition of Eqn. 1.5 ensures that the speed F goes to zero rapidly and minimizes the over-shoot effect. However, to be further accurate, we now follow the ideas in [17,18,4,12] and outline how additional constraints can be imposed on the surface motion.

1.3.1   Level set method

First, note that the shape model is represented implicitly as a particular level set of a function $\psi(\mathbf{x})$ defined in the image domain. As shown in section 2,

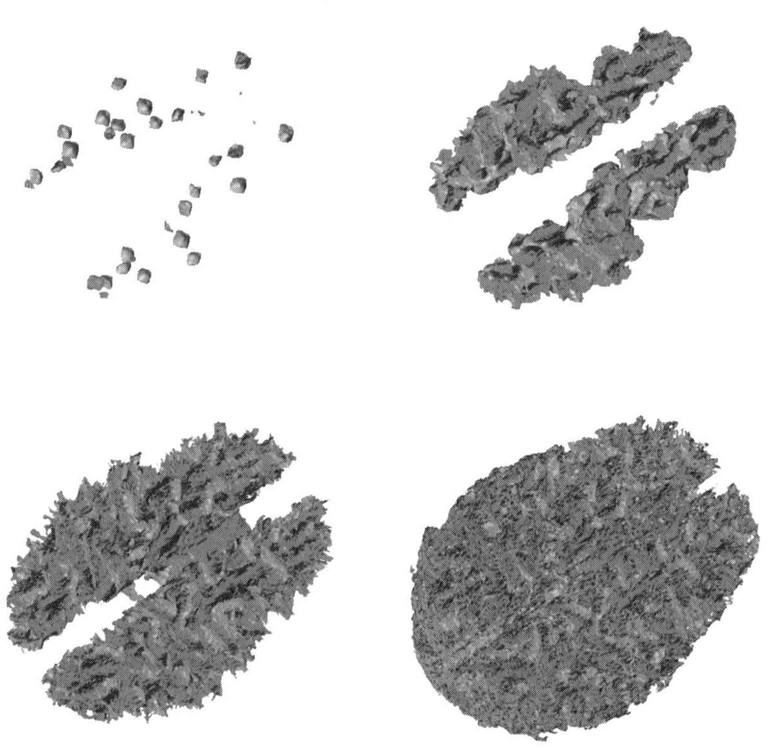

Fig. 1.2. Evolutionary sequence showing the brain reconstruction. Here we have rendered particular level sets of the function $T(x, y, z)$; the surfaces in the left-to-right top-to-bottom order correspond to the values $T(x, y, z) = 0.01, 0.125, 0.25, 0.75$.

Grid Size	Time to Load Speed File	Time to Propagate Surface	Total Time
$256 \times 256 \times 124$	8.61 secs	74.92 secs	83.53 secs

Fig. 1.3. Timing for Marching to T=0.75: Sun SPARC 1000

an evolution equation can be written for the function ψ such that it contains the motion of the surface embedded in it. Let the surface move under a simple speed law $F = 1 - \epsilon K$, where $K(\mathbf{x})$ is the curvature and $\epsilon > 0$. The constant component of F causes the model to seek object boundaries and the curvature component controls the regularity of the deforming shape. Geometric quantities like surface normal and curvature can be extracted from

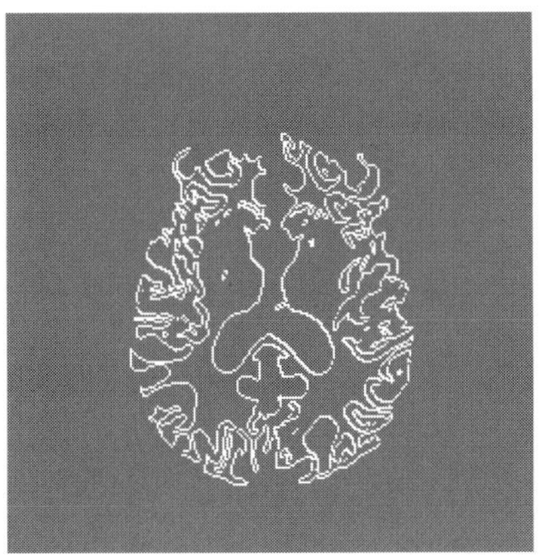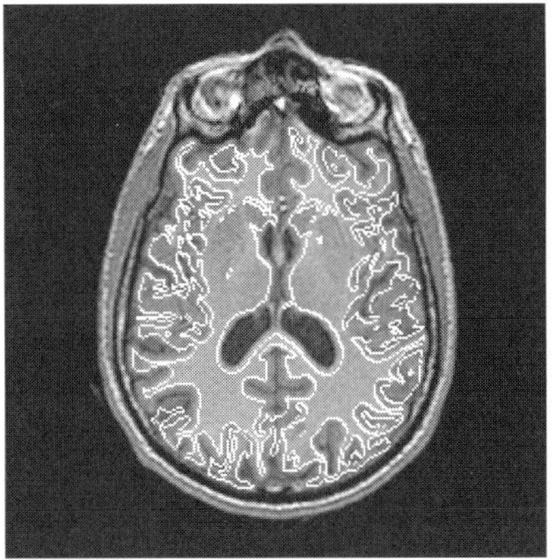

Fig. 1.4. We depict a slice of the brain surface superimposed on the corresponding image.

the higher dimensional function ψ; for example

$$K = \frac{\psi_{xx}\psi_y^2 - 2\psi_x\psi_y\psi_{xy} + \psi_{yy}\psi_x^2}{(\psi_x^2 + \psi_y^2)^{3/2}} \tag{1.6}$$

in $2D$ and in $3D$ the mean curvature is given by the expression

$$K = \frac{N_1 - 2N_2}{(\psi_x^2 + \psi_y^2 + \psi_z^2)^{3/2}}, \tag{1.7}$$

where $N_1 = \psi_{xx}(\psi_y^2 + \psi_z^2) + \psi_{yy}(\psi_x^2 + \psi_z^2) + \psi_{zz}(\psi_x^2 + \psi_y^2)$, and
$N_2 = \psi_{xy}\psi_x\psi_y + \psi_{yz}\psi_y\psi_z + \psi_{zx}\psi_z\psi_x$.

The driving force that molds the initial surface into desired anatomical shapes comes from two image-based terms. The first one is similar to Eqn. 1.5 and the second term attracts the surface towards the object boundaries; the latter term has a stabilizing effect especially when there is a large variation in the image gradient value. Specifically, the equation of motion is

$$\psi_t + g_I(1 - \epsilon K)|\nabla\psi| - \beta\nabla P \cdot \nabla\psi = 0. \tag{1.8}$$

where,

$$g_I(\mathbf{x}) = \frac{1}{1+ \mid \nabla G_\sigma * I(\mathbf{x}) \mid}. \tag{1.9}$$

The second term $\nabla P \cdot \nabla\psi$ denotes the projection of an (attractive) force vector on the surface normal. This force which is realized as the gradient of a potential field (see [4])

$$P(\mathbf{x}) = -|\nabla G_\sigma * I(\mathbf{x})|, \tag{1.10}$$

attracts the surface to the edges in the image; coefficient β controls the strength of this attraction.

In this work, we adopt the following two stage approach when necessary. We first construct the arrival time function using our marching algorithm. If a more accurate reconstruction is desired, we treat the final $T(\mathbf{x})$ function as an initial condition to our full model. In other words, we solve Eqn. 1.8 for a few time steps using explicit finite-differencing with $\psi(\mathbf{x}; t = 0) = T(\mathbf{x})$. This too can be done very efficiently in the narrow band framework [18,1]. Finally, the above initial condition is a valid one since the surface of interest is a particular level set of the final time function T.

1.4   Results

In this section, we present some shape recovery results from $2D$ and $3D$ medical images using the two-stage procedure we described in the previous section. We begin by defining seed points inside the region of interest; in most cases one mouse click will suffice. The value of $T(\mathbf{x})$ at these points is set to zero and the initial heap in order to start the marching method is constructed from their neighbors. We then employ the marching method to march until a fixed time or until the size of heap doesn't change very much between two successive time increments. This ends stage #1 of our scheme. We pass the final $T(\mathbf{x})$ function as the initial state to Eqn. 1.8 which is then solved for a few time steps. In $2D$, this whole procedure takes less than a second on a typical Sun SPARC workstation and to recover a $3D$ shape, the method executes in few tens of seconds.

First, we present some results in $2D$. In the first row of Fig. 1.5, we show a 256×256 image of the thoracic region along with the user-defined seed point inside the liver cross-section. The marching method is run until $T(x, y) = 0.90$; the second image depicts the level set $\{T = 0.75\}$. This function is then treated as the initial state to our full method, Eqn. 1.8, and the final shape, the level set $\{\psi = 0.75\}$, is shown in the last image. Notice that the recovered liver cross-section is both smooth and matches very closely with the perceived shape. In the second row of Fig. 1.5, we show the same sequence with the same parameters to reconstruct the shape of left ventricle from a different image. Finally, in the third row of the Fig. 1.5), we show the final shapes of left ventricle cross-sections from three other images. We recover the cell outlines from a large micrograph with varying contrast in the next example. These images are generated by using a counterstain to create a contrast between either the nuclei or the cell and the background. As shown in Fig. 1.6, the number of cells is very large and requires a completely automatic method to isolate them. Our computation starts from a single point in the background and using the two stage procedure described above, extracts the shapes of all the regions in the image. The next $2D$ example is from single particle reconstruction project in structural biology. The image shown in Fig. 1.7, is cropped from one of several hundred electron micrographs depicting many possible projections of a complex particle like the ribosome. The idea is

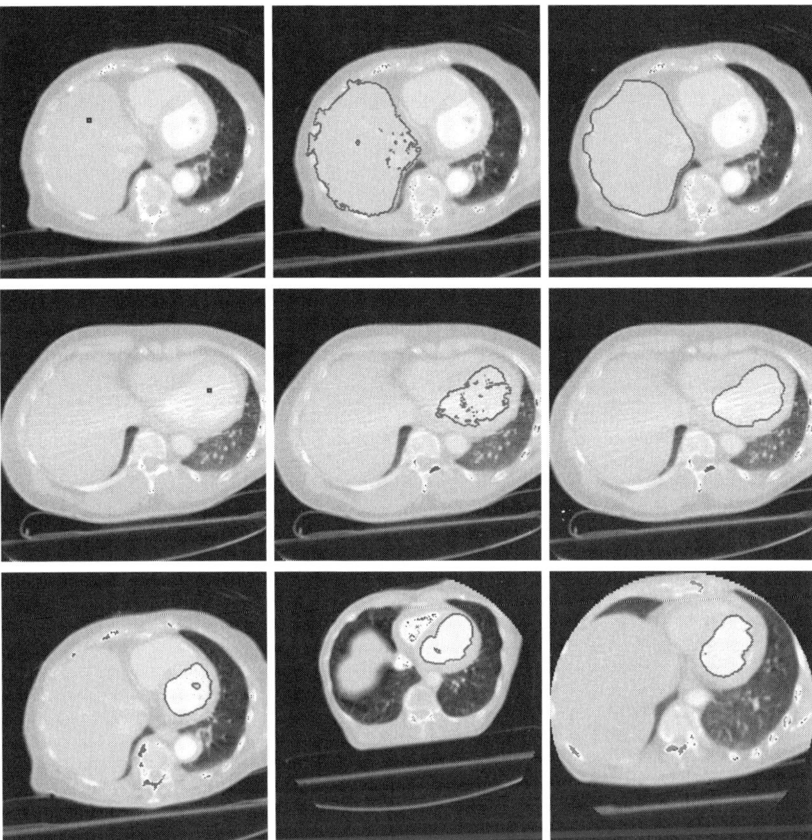

Fig. 1.5. $2D$ examples of our two-stage shape recovery scheme. From left-to-right in the first two rows we show (a) the initial mouse click, (b) the end of Stage # 1, and (c) the end of Stage #2. In the last row we show three more converged results.

to identify these particle projections that are typically smaller than 30-50 Å, and ultimately create a complete $3D$ description of it. The images are very noisy due in part to very low energy illumination requirement. The figure shows the final result of identifying the particle projections; the result has been post-processed to eliminate contours that are either too large or too small to be of value to subsequent stages of analysis.

In the next set of figures, we present examples in $3D$. Figure 1.8 shows the reconstruction of spleen from a $3D$ CT image of size $256 \times 256 \times 64$. We begin by initializing stage # 1 with a set of mouse clicks in the image domain; see the top two rows of Fig. 1.8. As we did before in Fig. 1.2, we render various isosurfaces of the final time function $T(x, y, z)$. Note that the shading model and colors used are purely artificial and have no relation to

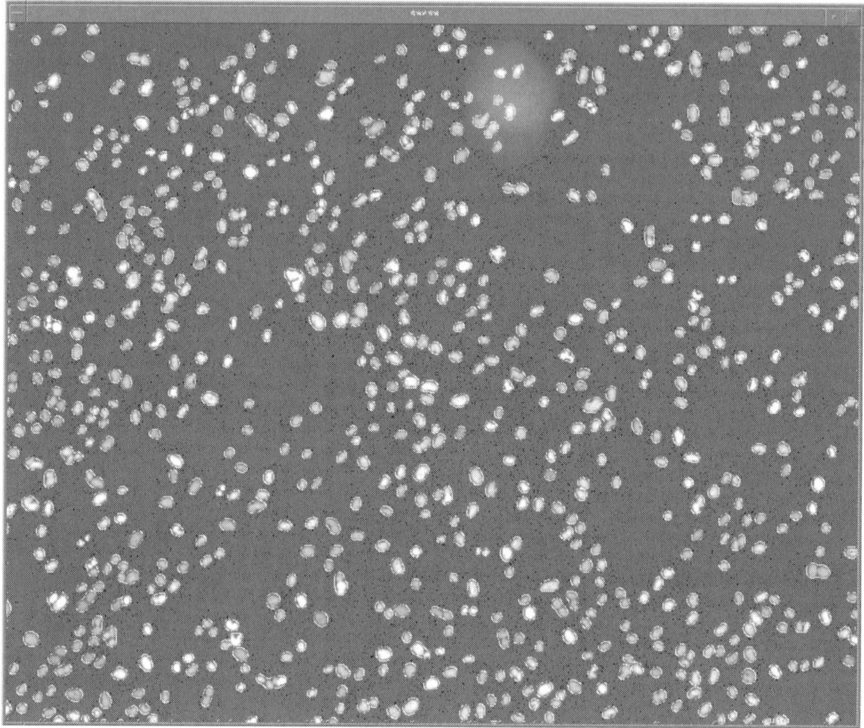

Fig. 1.6. Fully automated cell shape recovery from a large electron micrograph.

the real organ. The time function T is passed as an initial state to the level set shape recovery equation which is then solved for a few steps in a narrow-band around the level surface $\{\psi = 0.1\}$. The result is shown in the third row of Fig. 1.8. As shown in the figure, the level surface $\{T = 0.1\}$ that marks the end of stage # 1, is noisy and is stopped a little further away from the object boundary compared to the final reconstruction. This is because the speed function in Eqn. 1.5 falls to zero rapidly. To check the fidelity of the surface, we slice it parallel to the xy plane and superimpose the resulting contour on the corresponding image slice; see Fig. 1.9.

Next, in the top row of Fig. 1.10, we show two views of the heart chambers reconstructed from the same $3D$ data set as above. In the second row of Fig. 1.10, we recover the brain and the outer skin surface from $3D$ MR head data of Fig. 1.2. Note that the brain shape shown here is the result of applying a few steps of Eqn. 1.8 on the time surface shown in Fig. 1.2; the result is both closer to the true edge and regularized. In the third row of Fig. 1.10, we show the shapes of liver and the lung surfaces extracted from NIH's visual human data set. Finally, in Fig. 1.11, we superimpose these surfaces of the actual $3D$ data in order to access how well the reconstruction matches the true perceived edges in the image.

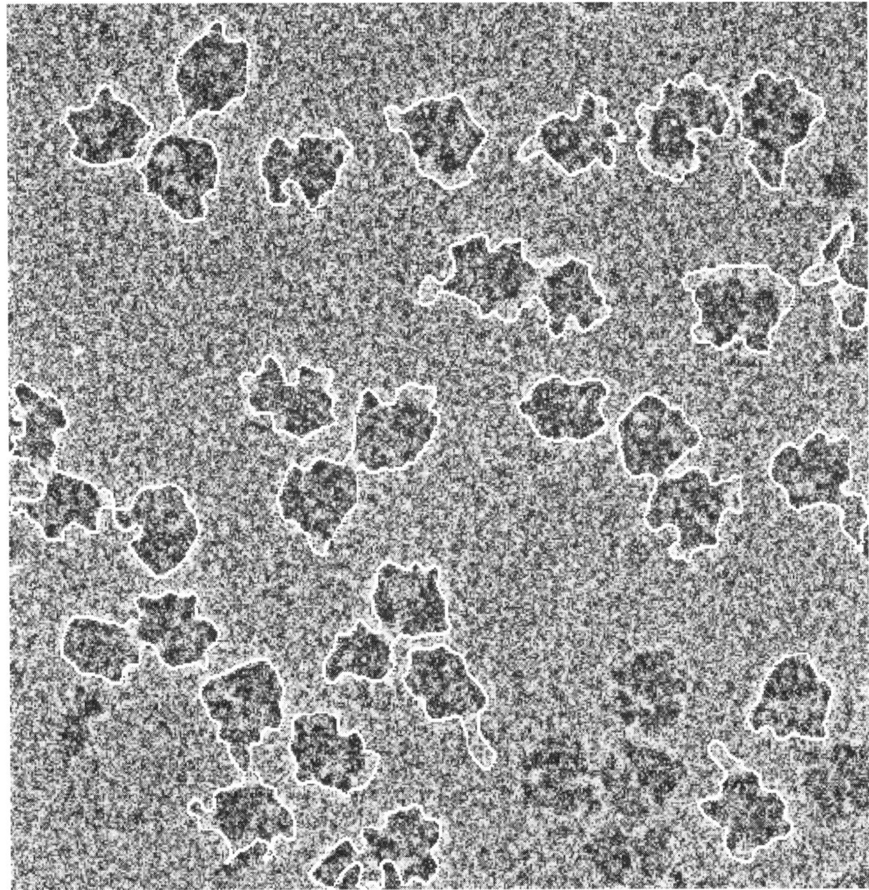

Fig. 1.7. Automatic particle selection from cryo-EM imagery.

Referenccs

1. D. Adalsteinsson and J. A. Sethian, "A fast level set method for propagating interfaces," *J. Comp. Phys.*, Vol. 118(2), pp. 269–277, May 1995.
2. D. Adalsteinsson, R. Kimmel, R. Malladi, and J. A. Sethian, " Fast marching methods for computing solutions to static Hamilton-Jacobi equations," submitted for publication, *SIAM Journal of Numerical Analysis*, January 1996.
3. V. Caselles, F. Catté, T. Coll, and F. Dibos, "A geometric model for active contours in image processing," *Numerische Mathematik*, Vol. 66(1), pp. 1–32, 1993.
4. V. Caselles, R. Kimmel, and G. Sapiro, "Geodesic snakes," *Proc. of ICCV*, MIT, Cambridge MA, June 1995.
5. V. Caselles, R. Kimmel, G. Sapiro, and C. Sbert, "Three-dimensional object modeling via minimal surfaces," *Proc. ECCV*, pp. 97–106, Cambridge, UK, April 1996.

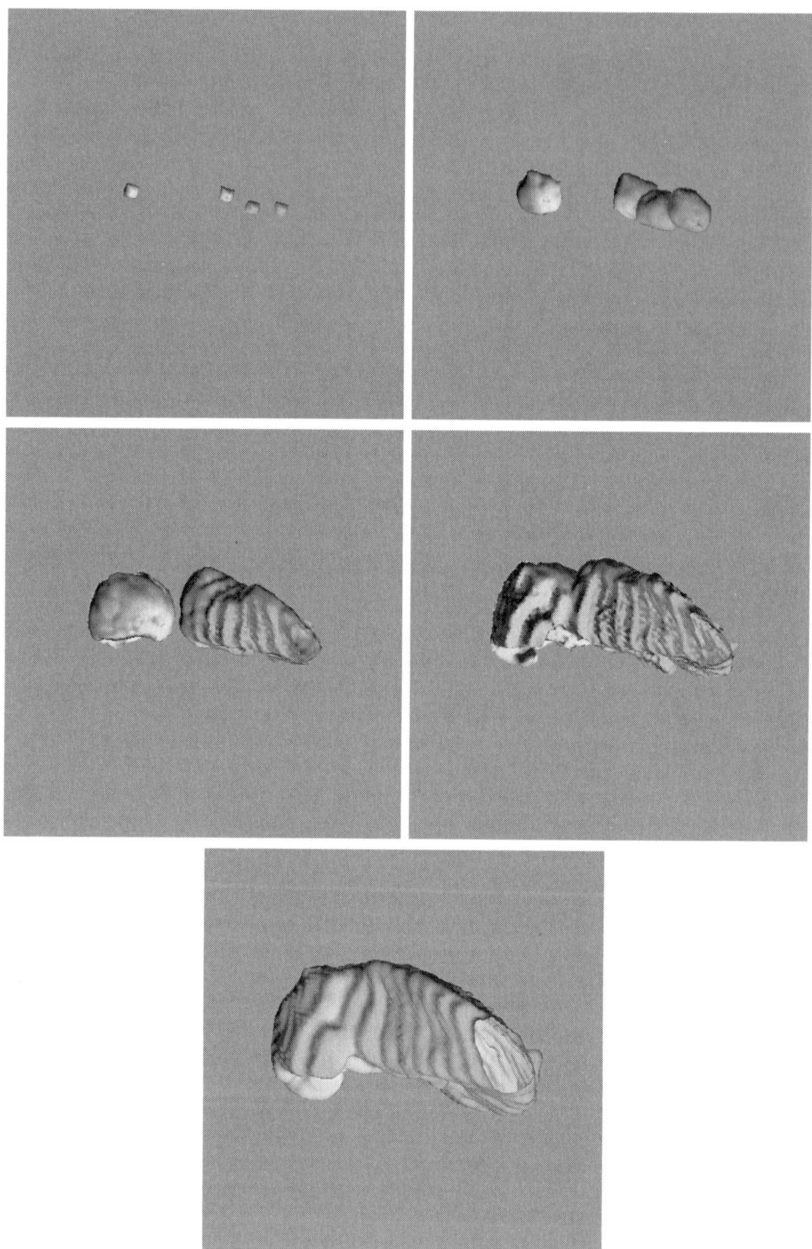

Fig. 1.8. The two-stage shape recovery in $3D$: the first four surfaces are the level sets $\{T(x, y, z) = 0.01\}$, 0.035, 0.07, and 0.10 respectively. This also marks the end of Stage #1. The result of solving the level set shape recovery equation for a few steps is shown in the final figure.

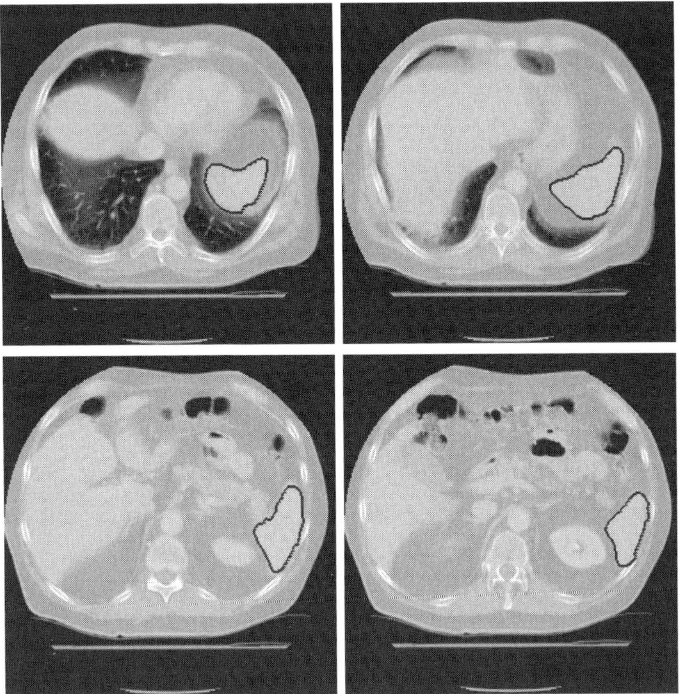

Fig. 1.9. Various slices of a CT image of the thoracic region and superimposed cross-section of the reconstructed spleen surface.

6. D. L. Chopp, "Computing minimal surfaces via level set curvature flow," *Journal of Computational Physics*, Vol. 106, pp. 77–91, 1993.

7. R. Goldenberg, R. Kimmel, E. Rivlin, and M. Rudzsky, "Fast active object tracking in color video," in *Proc. the 21 IEEE convention of the Electrical and Electronic Engineers in Israel*, Tel Aviv, April 2000.

8. Helmsen, J., Puckett, E.G., Colella, P., and Dorr, M., *Two new methods for simulating photolithography development*, SPIE 1996 International Symposium on Microlithography, SPIE, v. 2726, June, 1996.

9. M. Kass, A. Witkin, and D. Terzopoulos, "Snakes: Active contour models," *International Journal of Computer Vision*, Vol. 1, pp. 321–331, 1988.

10. S. Kichenassamy, A. Kumar, P. Olver, A. Tannenbaum, and A. Yezzi, "Gradient flows and geometric active contour models," *Proc. of ICCV*, MIT, Cambridge MA, June 1995.

11. R. Malladi and J. A. Sethian, "An $O(N \log N)$ algorithm for shape modeling," *Proc. Natl. Acad. Sci., USA*, Vol. 93, pp. 9389–9392, September 1996.

12. R. Malladi and J. A. Sethian, "Level set methods for curvature flow, image enhancement, and shape recovery in medical images," *Proc. of International Conference on Mathematics and Visualization*, H. C. Hege, K. Polthier (eds), pp. 255–267, Springer-Verlag, Berlin, Summer 1996.

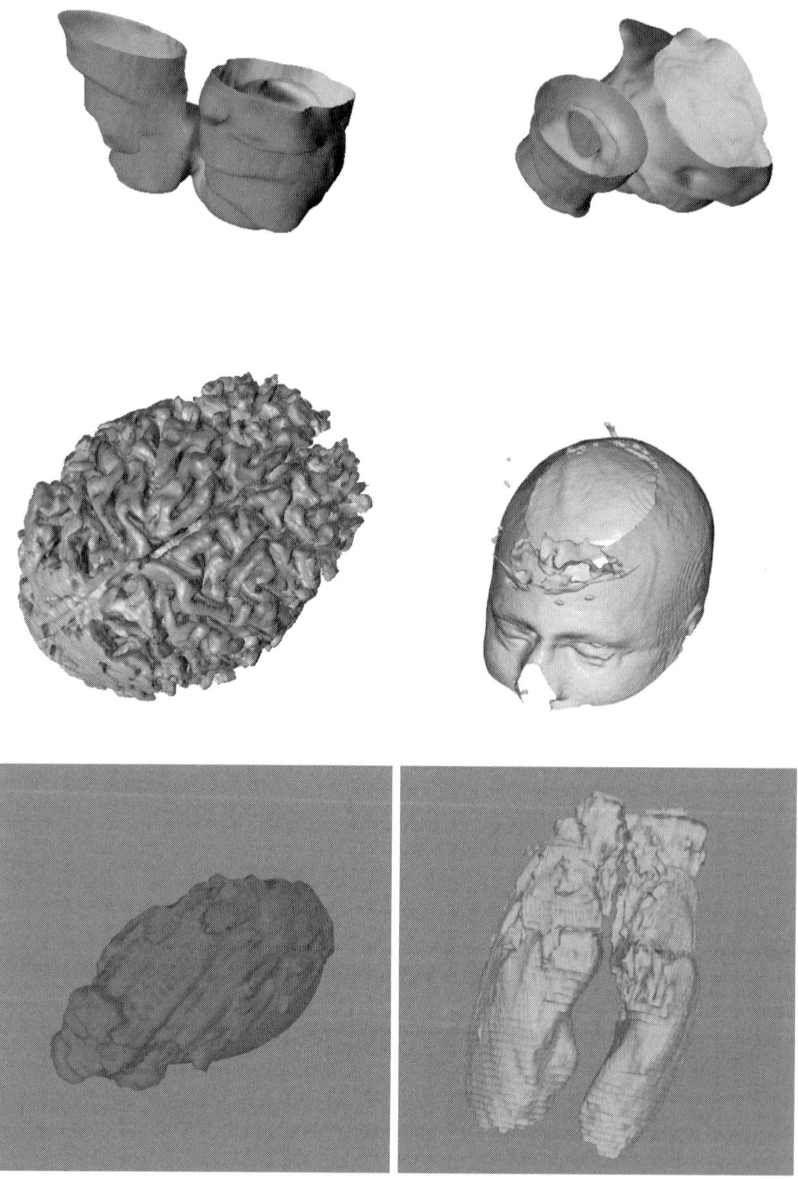

Fig. 1.10. More examples of $3D$ shape recovery.

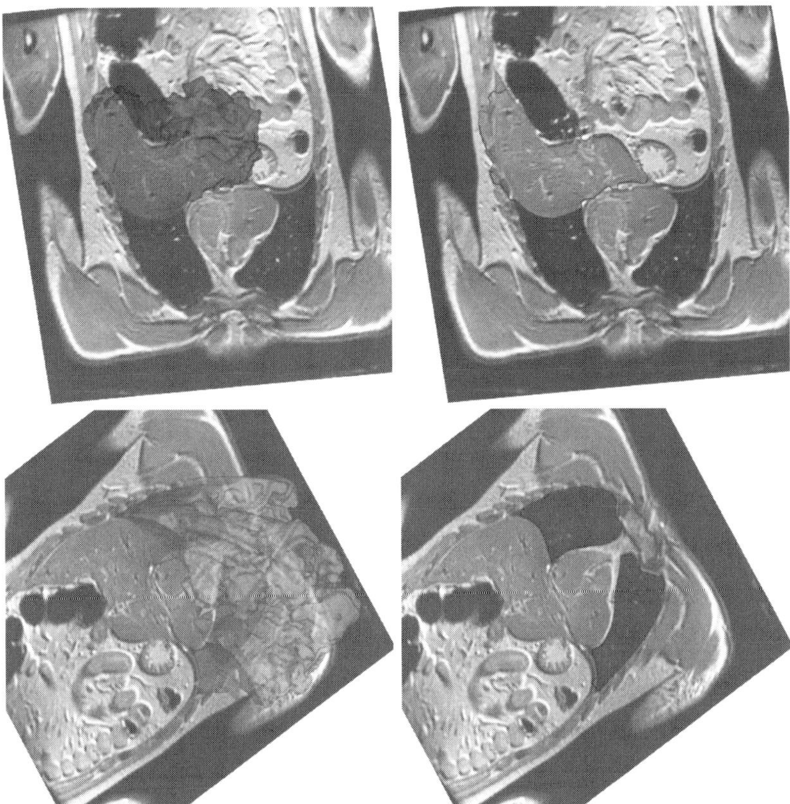

Fig. 1.11. $3D$ results superimposed on a particular $2D$ image slice.

13. R. Malladi and J. A. Sethian, "Image processing via level set curvature flow,"
Proc. Natl. Acad. Sci., USA, Vol. 92, pp. 7046–7050, July 1995.
14. R. Malladi and J. A. Sethian, "Image processing: Flows under Min/Max curvature and mean curvature," *Graphics Models and Image Processing*, Vol. 58(2), pp. 127–141, March 1996.
15. R. Malladi and J. A. Sethian, "A unified approach to noise removal, image enhancement, and shape recovery," *IEEE Transactions on Image Processing*, Vol. 5, No. 11, November 1996.
16. R. Malladi, J. A. Sethian, and B. C. Vemuri, "A topology-independent shape modeling scheme," in *Proc. of SPIE Conference on Geometric Methods in Computer Vision II*, Vol. 2031, San Diego, California, pp. 246–258, July 1993.
17. R. Malladi, J. A. Sethian, and B. C. Vemuri, "Evolutionary fronts for topology-independent shape modeling and recovery," in *Proceedings of Third European Conference on Computer Vision*, LNCS Vol. 800, pp. 3–13, Stockholm, Sweden, May 1994.
18. R. Malladi, J. A. Sethian, and B. C. Vemuri, "Shape modeling with front propagation: A level set approach," in *IEEE Trans. on Pattern Analysis and Machine*

Intelligence, Vol. 17, No. 2, pp. 158–175, Feb. 1995.

19. R. Malladi, R. Kimmel, D. Adelsteinsson, G. Sapiro, V. Caselles, and J. A. Sethian, "A geometric approach to segmentation and analysis of 3*D* medical images," *Proc. of IEEE/SIAM workshop on Mathematical Methods in Biomedical Image Analysis*, pp. 244–252, San Francisco, CA, June 1996; submitted to *CVIU*.

20. R. B. Milne, "An adaptive level set method," *Ph. D. Thesis*, Report LBNL-39216, Lawrence Berkeley National Laboratory, University of California, December 1995.

21. T. McInerney and D. Terzopoulos, "Topologically adaptable snakes," *Proc. ICCV*, Cambridge, MA, June 1995.

22. S. Osher and J. A. Sethian, "Fronts propagating with curvature dependent speed: Algorithms based on Hamilton-Jacobi formulation," *Journal of Computational Physics*, Vol. 79, pp. 12-49, 1988.

23. N. K. Paragios and R. Deriche, "A PDE-based level approach for detections and tracking of moving objects," in *Proceedings of ICCV'98*, pp. 1139–1145, Bombay, India, Jan. 1998.

24. N. K. Paragios and R. Deriche, "Coupled geodesic active regions for image segmentations: A level set approach," in *Proc. ECCV*, Dublin, Ireland, June 2000.

25. R. Sedgewick, *Algorithms*, Addison-Wesley Publ., 1988.

26. J. A. Sethian, "Curvature and the evolution of fronts," *Commun. in Mathematical Physics*, Vol. 101, pp. 487–499, 1985.

27. J. A. Sethian, "A marching level set method for monotonically advancing fronts," *Proc. Natl. Acad. Sci., USA*, Vol. 93(4), 1996.

28. J. A. Sethian, "A review of the theory, algorithms, and applications of level set methods for propagating interfaces," *Acta Numerica*, pp. 309–395, 1996.

29. Sethian, J.A., *Fast Marching Level Set Methods for Three-Dimensional Photolithography Development*, Proceedings, SPIE 1996 International Symposium on Microlithography, Santa Clara, California, June, 1996.

30. J. A. Sethian, *Level set methods: Evolving interfaces in geometry, fluid dynamics, computer vision, and material sciences*, Cambridge University Press, 1996.

31. J. Shah, "Recovery of shapes by evolution of zero-crossings," Tech. Report, Math. Dept, Northwestern University, Boston, MA, 1995.

32. N. Sochen, R. Kimmel, and R. Malladi, "From high energy physics to low level vision," Report LBNL-39243, Lawrence Berkeley Natl. Laboratory, Berkeley, August 1996; submitted to *IEEE Trans. Image Processing*, special issue on PDE and Geometry-Driven Diffusion in Image Processing and Analysis.

33. D. Terzopoulos, A. Witkin, and M. Kass, "Constraints on deformable models: Recovering 3D shape and nonrigid motions," *Artificial Intelligence*, Vol. 36, pp. 91–123, 1988.

34. Tsitsiklis, J.N., *Efficient Algorithms for Globally Optimal Trajectories*, IEEE Transactions on Automatic Control, Volume 40, pp. 1528-1538, 1995.

35. R. T. Whitaker, "Algorithms for implicit deformable models," *Proc. ICCV*, pp. 822–827, Cambridge, MA, June 1995.

2 A Geometric Model for Image Analysis in Cytology

C. Ortiz de Solorzano,[1] R. Malladi,[1] and S. J. Lockett[2]

[1] Lawrence Berkeley National Laboratory
   University of California, Berkeley CA 94720, USA
[2] SAIC-Frederick, Frederick MD 21702, USA

Abstract. In this chapter, we propose a unified image analysis scheme for 3D computer assisted-cytology. The goal is to accurately extract and classify the shapes of nuclei and cells from confocal microscopy images. We make use of a geometry-driven scheme for preprocessing and analyzing confocal microscopy images. Namely, we build a chain of methods that includes an edge-preserving image smoothing mechanism, an automatic segmentation method, a geometry-driven scheme to regularize the shapes and improve edge fidelity, and an interactive method to split shape clusters and reclassify them. Finally we apply our scheme to segmenting nuclei using nuclear membrane and whole cells using cell-surface related proteins.

2.1 Introduction

Determining where in a tissue or organ a particular molecular event occurs is a piece of valuable information not normally provided by most standard analytical methods in Biology. Although very informative, they only study a limited number of elements (e.g. genes, RNA's, expressed proteins, etc.) extracted from a 'sample' of cells which only partially represents the entire tissue or organ being analyzed. As a consequence, one must assume that what is seen or measured in one sample represents the behavior of the entire colony or organ. Quite often, this assumption falls short due to the inherent heterogeneity of any living tissue. For instance, the expression of a particular protein within a cell varies a great deal between different parts of a tissue, and even between neighboring cells within a particular region of the tissue. Therefore, the ability to do a per cell or per nucleus analysis of a particular molecular or cellular event, and then to do spatial statistical analysis of that event throughout the entire tissue or cell culture is a very important technical capability.

Individual cell analysis of a tissue sample can be achieved using Flow (FC)or Image Cytometry (IC). In FC, the tissue must be dissociated and the cells inserted in a one-cell wide water flow perpendicular to a laser-based detection system. This method, although very fast, can not account for any real 'geographical' heterogeneity, since the tissue has to be dissociated to obtain the linear cell flow. Image Cytometry, based on acquisition and analysis of microscopic images of thick tissue samples followed by computer-based delineation of cells and nuclei on the images -a process called segmentation- provides the desired geographical information.

Our initial $3D$ nuclei segmentation approach [30] is semi-automatic, in that it requires manual classification of the segmented objects. This permits correct segmentation of a high proportion of individual nuclei in intact tissue, with an accuracy similar to that of manual segmentation methods. However, the method needs improvements by way of better edge fidelity, especially for clusters of highly irregular nuclei and for nuclei with uneven DNA staining.

Encouraged by recent advances [22][23][24][25][40][2][6][36][26] in partial differential equation (PDE) based image analysis, we applied some of those methods to our confocal microscope image analysis. Starting with a general governing equation, we exploited its many interpretations, which include tasks such as edge-preserving image denoising and shape extraction and refinement. Various forms of our equation were then implemented using the level set [32] methods and the efficient narrow-band versions [1][22]. The flowchart in Fig. 2.1 shows the exact sequence of steps we used in order to process and analyze each $3D$ confocal microscope image.

The rest of this chapter is split into three sections; in Section 2.2 we introduce the geometric model, in Section 2.3 we summerize the work first published in Sarti *et al.* [37], and in Section 2.4 we follow the work of Ortiz de Solorzano *et al.* [31].

2.2 Geometric Model for Image Analysis

In this section, we introduce a geometric model; various forms of which are used in this paper to implement our image analysis procedures. The method relies on estimating the motion of curves and surfaces that move in the normal direction at a given speed. Given a hypersurface $\gamma(\mathbf{x})$ that is moving under speed $F(\mathbf{x})$, we adopt the level set equation to represent its motion [32] [38][39]. In other words, we embed the hypersurface as the zero level set of a higher dimensional function $\psi(\mathbf{x})$, and write the following equation of motion by following the chain rule:

$$\psi_t + F \mid \nabla\psi \mid = 0, \tag{2.1}$$

with a given initial condition $\psi(\mathbf{x}, t = 0) = \psi_0$.

This model of curve and surface motion has been applied to the problem of shape modeling in [21][8][22][24]. Imagine that one is given an image and the problem is to extract boundary descriptions of all the shapes implicitly present in it. The approach in [22] is one of using a trial shape that propagates in the image domain and molds itself into the desired boundary. The speed function used to control this shape recovery process is a combination of constant inflationary speed, a geometry dependent speed that regularizes the final result, and an image-dependent speed. Specifically, the equation of

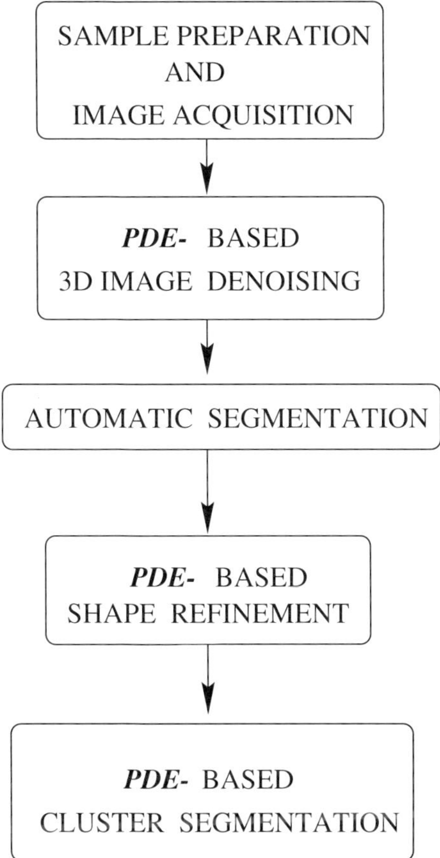

Fig. 2.1. Flowchart depicting the sequence of steps we undertake

motion is given by,

$$\psi_t + g(1 - \epsilon H) \mid \nabla \psi \mid = 0, \tag{2.2}$$

where g is a decreasing function of the image gradient and H is the mean curvature. An additional forcing term can be added to this equation to improve the accuracy in the presence of large variations in image gradient. This is often realized by advecting the surface along an image dependent vector field [9][24]; the force field is synthesized in such a way that it always points in the edge direction. With this change, our equation becomes

$$\psi_t + g(1 - \epsilon H) \mid \nabla \psi \mid -\beta \nabla g \cdot \nabla \psi = 0. \tag{2.3}$$

This equation is then solved with a user-defined initial condition. The key advantages of our geometric model over other shape recovery schemes is its topological adaptability, and its robust and fast real-time numerical implementations [25] on dense multi-dimensional data.

2.3   Segmentation of Nuclei

To obtain quantitatively accurate measurements of individual, intact nuclei, thick (> 20 micron) sections must be analyzed. This requires three-dimensional ($3D$) (confocal) microscopic image acquisition [41] and $3D$ image analysis. To allow the segmentation of nuclei, we label the tissue sections with a fluorescent DNA-binding counterstain that produces images with high intensity nuclear regions and low intensity non-nuclear (background) regions. Nuclear segmentation can then be achieved by either interactive or automatic algorithms. Interactive methods, based on drawing contours around nuclei in consecutive [11][33] or orthogonal [20] $2D$ slices provide the highest performance (defined as the fraction of nuclei correctly segmented) based on visual judgment of the results. However, they are slow and require intense human interaction, being practical only when just few nuclei must be analyzed.

Fully automatic algorithms [3][16], on the other hand, are faster, thus enabling the analysis of 100s of nuclei. Their performance is very high ($> 90\%$) when applied to specimens containing isolated or not too densely clustered nuclei, but decreases drastically for highly populated samples. Our method [30], combines the accuracy of interactive algorithms with the speed of the automatic approach, by introducing an interactive classification step that ensures accuracy with a very investment in interaction. In the following sections, we explain our basic segmentation approach along with some important improvements.

2.3.1   Sample preparation and microscopy

We segmented a variety of tissues: *Caenorhabditis elegans* embrios, normal human skin, normal human breast tissue, MCF7 cells (a human breast cancer cell line) grown in mice as a Xenograft, and on human breast biopsies of Invasive Carcinoma. All the samples were fixated with neutral buffered formalin, embedded in paraffin to preserve their morphology and sliced into 20 to 40 microns thick sections. The nuclear DNA was then stained with either Propidium Iodide (PI) or YO-PRO-1.

The tissue sections were imaged on two confocal microscopes: a Zeiss Laser Scanning Confocal Microscope 410 and a Biorad MRC-1000 confocal imaging system. The Zeiss system is equipped with an Axiovert 100 microscope, a x63 1,4 NA Plan-Apochromat oil-immersion objective lens, an Argon/Krypton (Ar/Kr) and a HeNe laser. The Biorad is built around a Nikon Diaphot 200 scope, with a 60x 1.4 PlanApo objective and an Ar/Kr laser. PI was excited with the 568 nm line of the (Ar/Kr)laser and imaged by filtering the emitted light with a 590 nm low-pass filter. YOPRO-1 was excited with the 633 nm line of the HeNe laser and detected using a 650 nm low-pass filter. Images we acquired as series of 2D optical slices 0.4 microns (avg.) apart, stored in ICS format [13] and transferred to a UNIX workstation for archival and analysis.

2.3.2 Image denoising

Image denoising aims at smoothing all the homogeneous regions that contain noise while retaining the location of the boundaries that define the shape of the represented structures. Traditional pre-processing algorithms (moving average, median and Gaussian filtering) reduce image noise at the expense of degrading the definition of the edges. Most of these methods assume a noise model that is too simplistic for biological imaging. In particular, the concentration variation of the fluorescence labeled molecules (in this case DNA) adds a de facto noise level that is virtually impossible to model.

Summarizing previously published data [37], we now show how we can use Eqn. (2.3) to denoise images. The basic idea is to delete the constant speed term and solve the equation with the noisy image as the initial condition, namely

$$\psi_t = gH \mid \nabla\psi \mid +\beta\nabla g \cdot \nabla\psi, \tag{2.4}$$

with $\psi(\mathbf{x}, t = 0) = I_0(\mathbf{x})$. The first term on the right of the above equation is a parabolic smoothing term and the second is a hyperbolic term. The proposed model is a selective smoothing of the $3D$ image, where the edges are preserved as much as possible. A contrast function g allows us to decide whether a detail is sharp enough to be kept. In our model, g is a smooth nonincreasing function of the initial image $I_0(x)$, namely

$$g = g(|\nabla(G(x) \otimes I_0(x))|) \tag{2.5}$$

where $G(x) =$ is a Gauss kernel and the symbol $\otimes$ denotes convolution.

In particular, $g(0) = 1$, $g(|\nabla(G(x) \otimes I_0(x))|) \geq 0$, and

$$\left(\lim_{|\nabla(G(x)\otimes I_0(x))|\to\infty} g(|\nabla(G(x) \otimes I_0(x))|) = 0 \right). \tag{2.6}$$

Typical forms of $g(|\nabla(G(x) \otimes I_0(x))|)$ are:

$$g(|\nabla(G(x) \otimes I_0(x))|) = e^{\frac{|\nabla(G(x)\otimes I_0(x))|}{\gamma}} \tag{2.7}$$

or

$$g(|\nabla(G(x) \otimes I_0(x))|) = \frac{1}{1 + \frac{|\nabla(G(x)\otimes I_0(x))|}{\gamma}}. \tag{2.8}$$

The smoothing works as follows: if $|\nabla(G(x) \otimes I_0(x))|$ is large, the flow is slow and the exact location of the edges will be retained. If $|\nabla(G(x)\otimes I_0(x))|$ is small then the flow tends to be fast thereby increasing the smoothing process. Notice that the filtering model reduces to mean curvature flow when $g(s) = 1$. A parameter we have to fix is the variance of the Gauss kernel. We note that the minimal size of the detail is related to the size of the Gauss kernel, which acts like a scale parameter. In fact the variance of $G_\sigma(x) = \frac{1}{C_\sigma}e^{-\frac{|x|^2}{4\sigma}}$ corresponds to the dimension of the smallest structures that have to be preserved. The second (hyperbolic) term in Eqn. (2.4) sharpens the edge information in the image; note that a similar observation was made in [34].

Now we present some results. Figure 2.3.2(a) is region of benign breast cancer, counterstained with PI for identification of the cell nuclei. The lower bilayer of nuclei are epithelial cells surrounding a duct. Figure 2.3.2(b) shows the result of solving Eqn. (2.4) using the image intensity values as an initial condition; Figure 2.3.2(c-d) shows the result of $3D$ edge-preserving smoothing on a portion of the confocal microscope image volume.

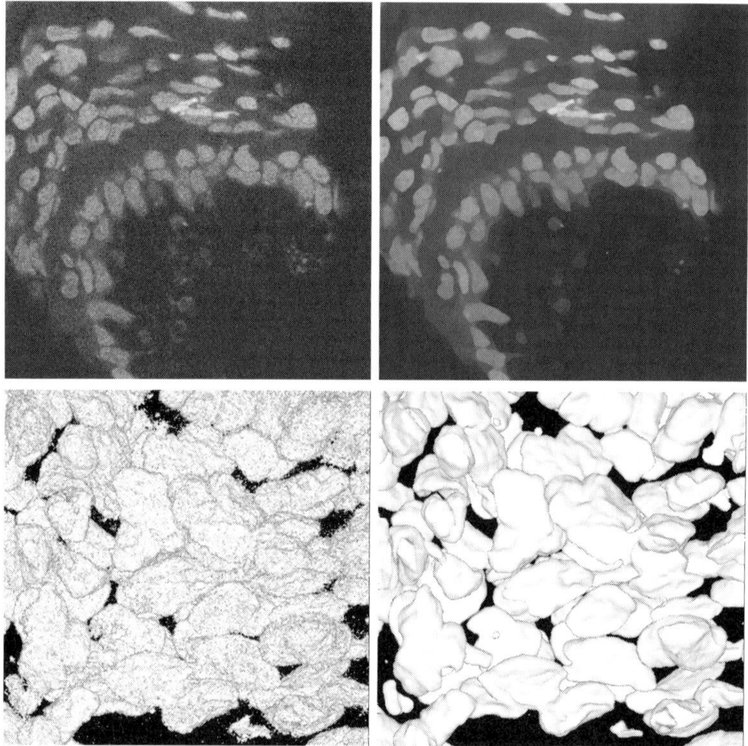

Fig. 2.2. $2D$ and $3D$ edge-preserving smoothing. (a) Top Left: $2D$ slice from the unfiltered image; (b)Top right: Filtering with $\beta = 1$ and $\sigma = 1$. (c)Bottom left: Surface rendering representation of the unfiltered volume. (d)Bottom Right: Filtering with $\beta = 1$ and $\sigma = 1$.

In [37] we validated our filter by comparing it with two other traditional filters used in confocal microscopy imaging (Median and Morphological Open-Close filter). The results, mesured by comparing the accuracy of the nuclear segmentation obtained after using each filtering scheme, show a clear improvement after applying our geometrically-driven filter.

2.3.3   Automatic segmentation

In this section, we briefly summarize previous work [30] on the automatic segmentation and classification of nuclear shapes. Our algorithm consists on following sequential steps:

First an adaptive gradient-weighted threshold is used to coarsely segment the images into DNA regions and background by taking advantage of the high contrast provided by the fluorescent nuclear stain.

Then the user visualizes and classifies each segmented object. The options are: the object is a nucleus, a cluster of nuclei or debris. To assist the user in classifying the objects, we developed a $3D$ visualization program: DAta VIsualization aNd Computer Interaction (DaVinci). DaVinci (Figure 2.3) creates a 3D surface rendering of the objects, which is displayed along with quantitative information about the rendered object. A variety of interaction tools (zooming, intersection of the rendered surface with $2D$ slices from the original $3D$ image, rotation, surface opacity control, etc.) helps the user to classify the objects.

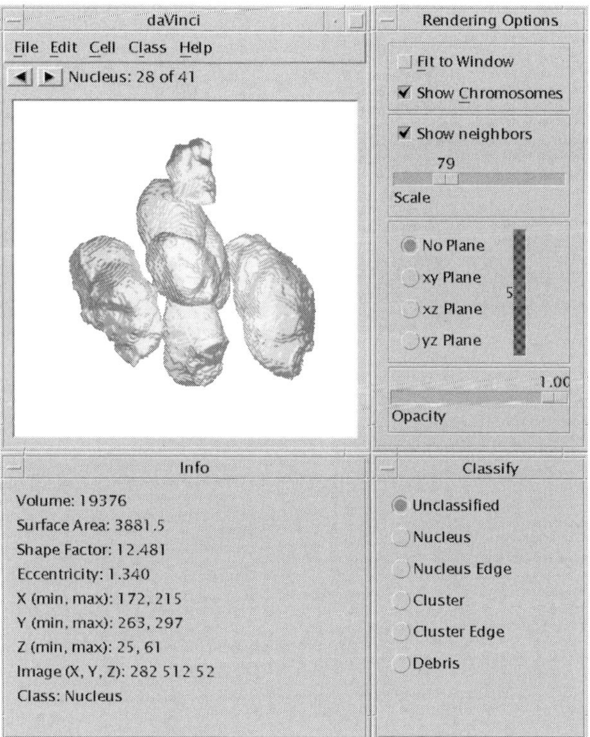

Fig. 2.3. DaVinci User Interface. (1) Top Left Panel: 3D graphics window showing some nuclei; (2) Top Right: Surface rendering options (3) Bottom Left: Quantitative Object Information; (4) Bottom Right: Object Classification Panel.

The objects classified as clusters are then divided into sub-components using a sequence of automatic algorithms: First the peaks of the Vector Distance Transform (VDT) of the cluster's binary mask are calculated. These peaks are individual markers of the nuclei that make up the cluster and will be used as the starting points in the following step. Then a watershed algorithm is applied to the inverse of either the VDT or the original grayscale image to find surfaces between nuclei in the cluster. The new objects thus obtained are then classified by the user. Incorrectly divided individual nuclei can then be merged.

The algorithm was tested on 2500 nuclei from five different types of samples that covered a range of segmentation difficulty levels. Specimens of non-densely clustered and approximately spherical nuclei could be easily segmented (99% of nuclei were correctly segmented based on visual verification). In specimens where nuclei were more clustered and variable in shape, performance deteriorated. For normal appearing human breast 90% of the nuclei could be segmented, but the percentage was lower for cancerous tissue. However, the main point to emphasize about the performance is that while not all nuclei in a specimen were segmented, the inclusion of the visual classification step meant that it was known which nuclei were correctly segmented and which were not.

Limitations of the current method We identified two main sources of error in the described segmentation method: (1) surface noise, which produces spurious peaks in the VDT image, causing inappropriate division surfaces by the Watershed algorithm; (2) the existence of unstained holes inside the nuclei that causes individual nuclei to be divided (oversegmentation).In the following sections, we explain how we used our unified geometric image denoising/enhancing scheme to address these two problems.

2.3.4   Shape refinement

As shown in Figure 2.4(a), the resulting surfaces from our automatic segmentation algorithm can be quite coarse with a lot of "voxelization". This is due to the fact that the thresholding-based segmentation creates a binary representation of the surface that either includes or excludes a given point as being in or out of the surface. This process produces an erroneous representation as the shape boundaries shown may be a little away from the true edges. We wish to correct this by refining the shapes using the geometrical flow introduced in previous sections. As we will show, the flow-based equation also makes it possible to represent the final surface with a sub-grid accuracy that is not possible with a threshold-based segmentation. To this end, let us revisit Eqn. (2.3), from the geometrical point of view of achieving boundary detection.

Assume that the surface $\mathcal{S}$ is a particular level set of a function $\psi :
[0, a] \times [0, b] \times [0, c] \rightarrow R$. In other words, $\mathcal{S}$ is a set of points at which

the function ψ is equal to a given constant. The embedding function ψ can therefore be considered as an implicit representation of the surface $\mathcal{S}$.

It is easy to prove that if a surface $\mathcal{S}$ evolves according to

$$\mathcal{S}_t = F\mathcal{N} \tag{2.9}$$

where $\mathcal{N}$ is the unit inward normal and F is a real function, then the level set function ψ obeys the following evolution rule

$$\psi_t = F|\nabla\psi|; \tag{2.10}$$

see [32][38] for details.

Our first objective is to produce a smoother representation of the surface using the above equation. In order to smooth a surface, we can let the speed F be equal to its mean curvature H. The flow decreases the total curvature and has the property of "smoothing out" all the high curvature regions on the surface, i.e. local variations [14]. However, this flow will also destroy useful surface features if run too long. One of the main issues concerning this flow is if there is a stopping criterion for an optimal shape refinement. Several methods have been proposed in the past, one of them adds a term to force the solution to remain close to the initial data [29], another method proposed by the the authors in [23] uses a scale dependent stop condition implemented via a $\min - \max$ curvature flow. In the present context, the stop condition is given by the g function. So, the surface moves according to the equation

$$\mathcal{S}_t = gH\mathcal{N}. \tag{2.11}$$

Our second objective is to steer the surface closer to the "true" edges in order to produce a better reconstruction. So, we rewrite Eqn. (2.3) without the constant speed term here:

$$\psi_t - gH\,|\,\nabla\psi\,| - \beta\nabla g \cdot \nabla\psi = 0, \tag{2.12}$$

where β is a non-zero constant. The first term smoothes the surface while keeping it close to the edges and the second term, $\beta\nabla g \cdot \nabla\psi$, attracts the surface closer to the edge map. The initial condition $\psi(\mathbf{x}, t = 0)$ is given by the signed distance function of the binary image obtained from a rough segmentation. The result of applying this flow on a coarse binary segmentation is shown in Figure 2.4.

2.3.5   Removal of unstained image regions

As mentioned earlier, the structure of a cluster is not always compact because it can contain several unstained regions (holes) inside. We can eliminate the holes by performing a *closing* operation, in the sense of the mathematical morphology, by a flow that provides sequentially a *dilation* and an *erosion*

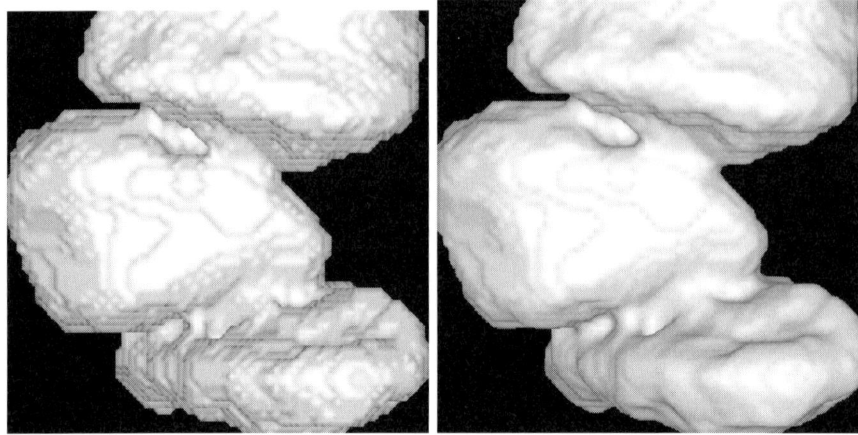

Fig. 2.4. Shape refinement; (a) Left: Zero level set of the signed distance function computed on the rough segmentation of a cluster of cells, and (b) Right: Geometric segmentation with $\beta = 1$ and $\sigma = 1$

effect. In the context of level set flow, the *closing* operation is achieved by considering two flows, $F = 1$ to obtain *dilation* and subsequently $F = -1$ for *erosion*.

In practice however, the *dilation* operation has to be performed carefully to avoid the merger of two close but distinct clusters, thus further complicating the problem. For that reason, we use a more sophisticated flow that eliminates the holes and is bounded by the convex hull of the original cluster. Specifically, the flow is given by

$$\psi_t = \min(H, 0.0)|\nabla \psi|. \tag{2.13}$$

This flow in $2D$ has been used recently in [23] in the context of image denoising and for surface smoothing in [24]. We have simply replaced the Euclidean curvature that was used for $2D$ image processing with the mean curvature in $3D$. The main feature of the flow is that it allows the inward concave regions to grow outwards, while suppressing the motion of the outward convex regions. Thus the evolving shape always remains inside the convex hull. The holes are thus subject to a mean curvature flow while the outer shape converges to its convex hull. In Figure 2.5 we show an example of hole elimination via $\min(K, 0)$ flow in a cropped sample of a nuclear cluster.

We notice from Figure 2.5 that hole elimination sometimes compromises the shape detail. In other words, the cell shapes stray away from high image gradients. We amend the loss in accuracy by solving our shape refinement equation, i.e. Eqn. (2.3), for a few time steps. Note that the image based component in the equation – the g function – is computed from the enhanced image. This procedure results in a cluster that is devoid of any holes and

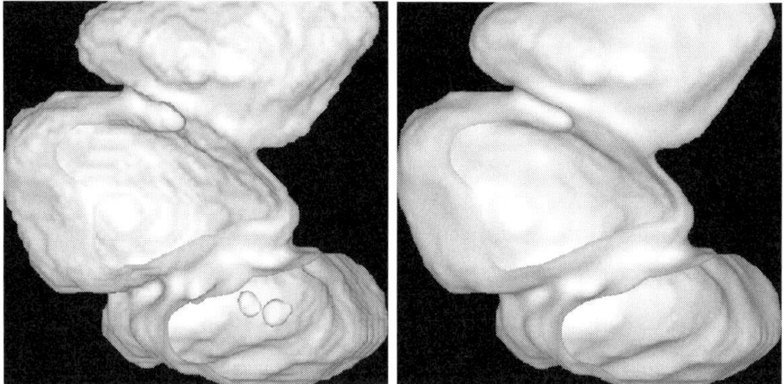

Fig. 2.5. Hole elimination. (a) Left: zero-level set of the refined shape. The volume has been cropped to reveal two internal holes. (b) Right: The shape after 10 iterations of the min flow. The holes disappear, but the shape looses detail.

close to the "true" edges present in the image; the shape after this step is shown in Figure 2.6.

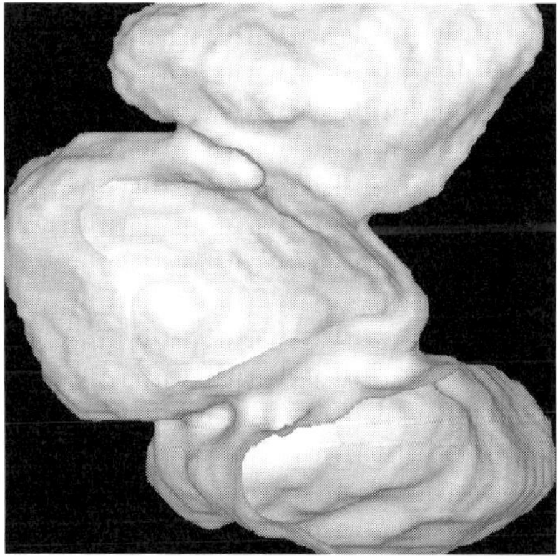

Fig. 2.6. The refined shape without holes after the geometric flow processing.

Multiple interface flow After the hole removal and shape refinement we can proceed to shrink the cluster until single nuclei emerge as topologically distinct objects. The main point of this section is how to grow them back to their original shape while maintaining their distinct identity. If we propagate the individual (nucleus) shape models according to Eqn. (2.3), they will be attracted to image edges but will merge into a cluster upon colliding with each other. That is exactly the behavior we wish to avoid. Instead, we would like the individual shapes to grow and segment the nuclear shapes, touch in areas where there is not enough delineating image gradient information, but never merge.

A similar problem arises when one tries to study the motion of multiple interfaces propagating in the same domain [39]. We follow the same idea here in order to build a scheme that moves shapes in a distinct manner. First, we build a separate level set function for each shape. Next, each shape is advanced to obtain a trial value for each level set function with the following geometrical flow

$$\frac{\partial \phi_i}{\partial t} = \nabla(g(|\nabla I_0|)\nabla \frac{\nabla \phi_i}{|\nabla \phi_i|}),$$ (2.14)

where ϕ_i is the level set function for the i-th shape. If two regions collide based on the trial function values, the value of the actual function is changed by considering the values of other level set functions. Merger can be avoided by a simple max operator. Further details can be found in [39].

We now present the result of cluster reclassification. Figure 2.6 shows the initial cluster (without holes) that we know from visual inspection contains three nuclei merged into one. Figure 2.7(a) is the result of shrinking the shape until it splits into three separate parts. These shapes are then evolved separately under the same image based g function using the multiple interface update rules; the result is shown in Figure 2.7(b). The three shapes shown in different colors segment three distinct nuclei.

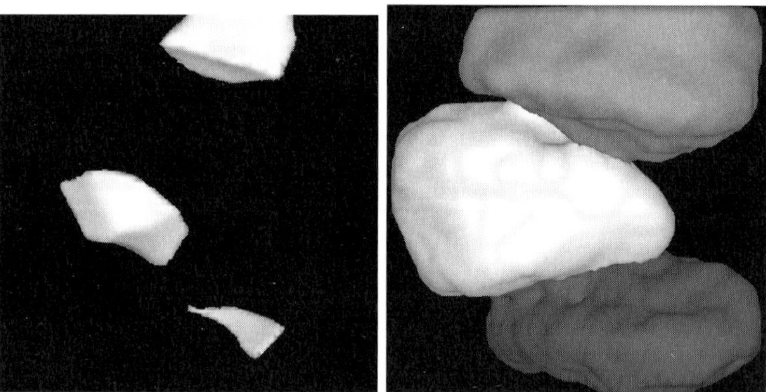

Fig. 2.7. The refined clusters after processing with the multiple interface flow. (a)Left: three distinct shapes after the *erode* operation. (b)Right: three different cells have been recognized and segmented.

2.4 Segmentation of Nuclei and Cells Using Membrane-Related Protein Markers

The success of the algorithms described above relies on the existence of background areas between the nuclei. Howeer, this does not happen in specimens with nuclei densely clustered or morphologically abnormal.

For those cases we have explored an alternate avenue to DNA stain based nuclear segmentation. It makes use of lamin, which is a protein located in the nuclear lamina, a protein mesh that underlies the inner membrane of the nuclear envelope. We can use fluorochrome-tagged antibodies against lamin, to obtain 2D or 3D (confocal) images where a detectable signal between neighboring nuclei nicely delimits the extent of each nucleus.

Since the segmentation problem is conceptually similar, we also want to segment whole cells to be able to quantify the expression of cytoplasmically localized proteins and mRNAs. For this we use cell surface protein markers. We believe that the use of cell surface markers is the only approach to whole-cell segmentation because cells always touch each other in solid tissue, being therefore "inherently clustered". To stain the surface we used antibodies against integrins, which are a family of cell-surface transmembrane proteins that facilitate cell-cell and cell-extracellular matrix interaction [7]. Specifically, we used alpha-6 (a6) and beta-1 (b1), because of its ubiquitous expression: it has been localized on almost all epithelial cell types as well as the endothelial cells of capillaries and in mast cells [18].

Our segmentation approach, explained in detail in [31], is based on the Geometric Model already introduced in this chapter. Our method first requires finding an internal seed that uniquely identifies each cell/nucleus in the image. Then each seed's surface is dilated until it aligns with the nuclear lamina or cell membrane surface.

2.4.1 Sample preparation and microscopy

We used both cell cultures and mouse mammary tissue. The cell culture was composed of HMT-3522 S1-50 human immortalized mammary epithelial cells (HMECs), propagated as monolayers in chamber slides. The tissue sections were taken from nulliparous mouse mammary gland, fresh frozen in embedding medium, fixed in methanol and sectioned. For nuclear lamina staining, we used mouse IgG1 and anti-laminB antibodies and secondary anti-mouse IgG1 FITC-conjugated antibody. For cell surface detection we used FITC conjugated alpha-6 or beta-1 antibodies.

Confocal images from cultured cells specimens were acquired using our Laser Scanning Confocal Microscope 410 The specimens were excited using the 488 nm. line of the Ar/Kr laser. The resolution of the images was close to the theoretical maximum (0.2 mm in the lateral (x, y) direction, 0.5 mm in the axial (z) direction). The images had an average of 40 z-sections and were manually selected to contain clusters of cells. Images were stored in the

ICS image format and transferred to a UNIX workstation for archiving and analysis. 2D images from a6 or b1 integrin stained tissue sections were imaged on an Axioplan Microscope (Carl Zeiss Inc., Thornwood, NY, USA), using a 40x, 0.75 NA Plan Neofluar objective lens (Zeiss), a 100W halogen lamp (Osram, Germany). Images were stored in TIFF format.

2.4.2   Segmentation

We'll describe how the algorithm works in 2D, although it is readily extendible to 3D:

First the algorithm finds a single seed inside each nucleus or cell. A seed is any closed area of the image entirely within the boundaries of its nucleus or cell. Our seed-finding method is inspired in the Hough Transform algorithm [4]. A full description of the method can be found in [30].

After seeds have been found, the boundary of each seed is moved until it aligns with the enclosing nucleus or cell, As described by the surface staining. This is done by solving the equation of the movement of the boundary from the initial position to that where it aligns with the surface of the nucleus or cell. We allow the boundary to move only in the normal direction, at a speed that depends on a force term $F(\mathbf{x})$ which is tuned to local characteristics of the boundary and to the properties of the original image. The particular details of the force term are described below. Once again, the equation that describes the movement of the curve is the general Eqn. 2.1, with a given initial condition which we chose to be the distance transform $d(\mathbf{x})$ of the seed $\psi(\mathbf{x})$, assigning negative distances for pixels inside the evolving object and positive distances for pixels outside it. The level zero curve $\psi(\mathbf{0}, \mathbf{t} = \mathbf{T})$ holds the position of the evolving boundary at any time point T. The rest of level sets are iso-distance curves $\psi(\mathbf{d}, \mathbf{t} = \mathbf{T})$, which contain all pixels located a distance d from the level set 0 at a given time T. We can see the evolution of the function as the evolution of a front of iso-distance surface. Thereafter we will use the term front to refer to this function.

The equation of the movement of $\psi(x)$ is solved using finite differences following an iterative scheme. Moving the front m steps is equivalent to calculating $\psi(\mathbf{d}, \mathbf{t} = \mathbf{m}\delta\mathbf{t})$ for all the pixels in the image. The evolution of the seed's boundary is defined by those pixels (i,j) in which $\psi_{i,j}(\mathbf{x}) = 0$ after m iterations of the algorithm, being δt the unit (quantum) movement per iteration. δt is an important parameter, since it determines the speed of the movement. If δt is too large the front will never converge to an stable solution, by voiding the effect of the force term. If δt is too small, errors do not arise, but the front evolves very slowly, with the consequent computational and time cost. Our approach to select δt is empirical. Once a value has been found appropriate for a given image, it can then be used for similar images. To reduce computation time, we used a narrow band method [39] that consists of updating the front only for those pixels located within a distance $d_{m}ax$ of the level set 0. This approach substantially reduces computation time by not updating the position of the front in areas which are far away from the zero level set. To keep consistency, the distance transform has to be rebuilt after several narrow band iterations. In our case we rebuilt it every 10 iterations, since we found that number a good tradeoff between computation time and accuracy.

If an image contains n nuclei, each seed is embedded in an independent function $\psi^i, (1 \leq i \leq n)$ which is moved independently of the other fronts. In order to prevent the fronts from crossing when they are expanding, their movement is limited by the position of the other fronts. Accordingly, every time a front is moved one step, the outcome is considered as a trial function. The final movement of the front is computed as the maximum between the value trial function and the value of the other fronts.

$$\psi^i_{m+1} = max\{\psi^i_{m+1(trial)}, \psi^j_m\}, 1 \leq j \leq n, i \neq j \qquad (2.15)$$

Sequence of flows To find the external side of the surfaces, we devised a sequence of flows which is described in the following sections, their effect being also illustrated on synthetic images (see Figures 2.8 and 2.9) which resemble the type of images that we want to segment. Figure 2.8(c) shows the initial seeds, which correspond to the zero level sets of $\psi^i_0, (1 \leq i \leq 3)$ at time zero.

Flow 1. Initial expansion The initial flow moves the front towards the internal side of the surface. It follows a particularization of the general Eqn. (2.3), in which the first term g effectively attracts the surface towards areas of the image with high gradient. This is done through the non-linear gradient function g which has the form of a familiar function used for denoising (Eq.2.7). The effect of g is to speed up the flow in those areas where the image gradient is low ($g \approx 1$) and slow it down where there is high gradient ($g \approx 0$). The parameter a determines the sensitivity of the flow to the gradient.

The effect of g is modulated by the second term $(1 - \epsilon H)$ which contains an inflationary term $(+1)$, enhanced or opposed by a curvature term (ϵH) that regularizes the surface by accelerating the movement of those parts of the surface that are behind the average of the front (and therefore have a negative curvature) and slowing down the advanced parts of the flow (parts with positive curvature). The parameter ϵ determines the strength of the regularization: a low ϵ allows creating or maintaining sharp corners on the fronts, while a high value will smooth out front irregularities. In the extreme case it will result in only circular objects. In practice an intermediate value of ϵ was chosen so that concavities in nuclear and cell borders were preserved, but bright spots from punctate staining, small gaps in the staining and noise were smoothed over.

The third term in (2.3), $\beta \nabla g$ is a parabolic term that enhances the edge effect, once an edge is reached due to the effect of the first two terms. This term aligns all the level sets with the ideal gradient, which would be a perfect step function, centered at the point of maximum gradient in the original image. Due to the gradient, the front slows down almost to a stop when it reaches the inner face of the nuclear surface. This can be used as the stop condition for the flow when the algorithm is run in unsupervised way. It can be implemented by checking the area or volume increase after each iteration, and setting a minimum threshold of volume change that, when reached, will interrupt the flow. Otherwise, a conservatively high number of iterations can be done that will ensure that the front will always reach the internal side of the stained surface. The result of this initial flow can be seen in 2.9(b). The flow described underestimates the nuclear shape, although it makes subsequent flows independent from the size or shape of the initial seeds. The purpose of the following flows is to correct for this under estimation.

The values of the parameters used in this flow, γ, β, ϵ, and δt were determined empirically. In our experience, a given set of parameters can be used for images with a broad range of image characteristics (gradient, noise level, etc.), as will be shown below. Varying the parameters or the image properties alters the speed of the segmentation (how fast the front converges to the final position) but not its accuracy.

Flow 2. Free expansion The second flow detaches the front from the inner surface of the surface, allowing it to freely expand independently from the gradient of the original image. The equation that describes the movement is:

$$\psi_t + \mid \nabla \psi \mid = 0 \tag{2.16}$$

Under this flow, the only limit to the expansion of a front is the position of the other fronts. Therefore, the expansion is allowed only for a number of steps that ensure that all the flows move beyond the outer surface. The number of steps can be empirically determined based on the membrane width. The result can be seen in 2.9(c).

Flow 3. Surface wrapping Finally, the surface must be moved inwards until it finds the external side of the stained surface. To do this we use the flow:

$$\psi_t - g(-1 - \epsilon H) \mid \nabla \psi \mid = 0. \tag{2.17}$$

which is similar to Eq. 2.3, but with a negative advection value, which moves the front inwards, and with the function g now depending on the intensity alone of the image, and not on its gradient.

$$g(\mid (G(x) \otimes I_0(x)) \mid) = e^{\frac{-\mid (G(x) \otimes I_0(x)) \mid}{\gamma}} \tag{2.18}$$

The last term in Eq. 2.3 is also removed. The effect of this flow is an inward movement opposed by high intensity values, as those represented by the maximum intensity of the stained lamina. The result is shown in Figure 2.9(d).

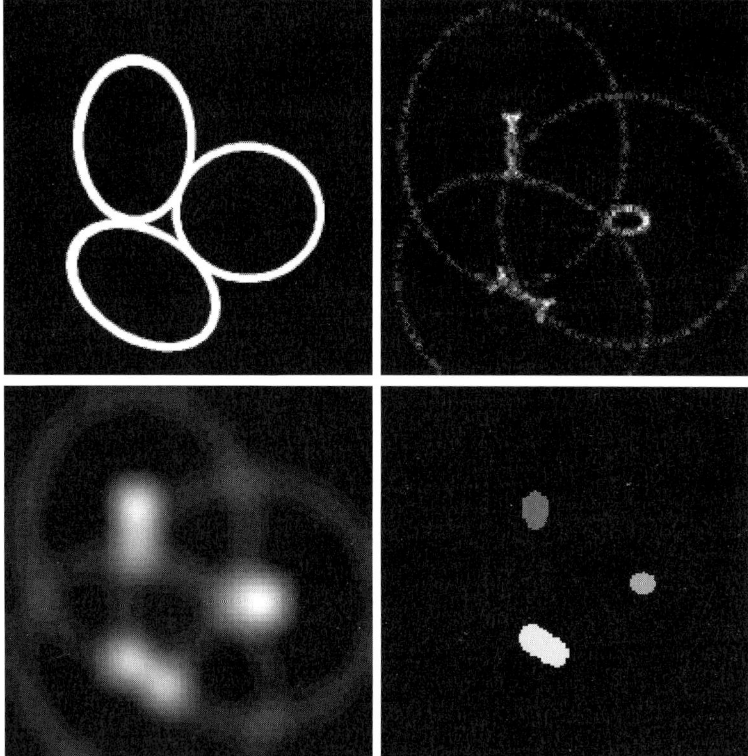

Fig. 2.8. Nuclear segmentation using a computer generated image. (a) Top left: simulation of a cluster of three surface stained nuclei. (b) Top right: Hough Transform of (a), where gradients in the original image are projected using and estimate of the object size. (c) Bottom left: Gaussian filtered version of (b). (d) Bottom Left: Final seeds obtained using a morphological peak detection algorithm.

The characteristics of the staining of the cellular surface using a6b1 integrins are similar to those of the nuclear staining using lamin antibodies. Therefore for segmenting whole cells we used the same sequence of flows, with identical parameters as the ones used for the image in 2.8. Figure 2.10 shows a computer model which represents a group of cells forming a structure that resembles a duct in mammary tissue. 2.10(a) is the original image with the seeds interactively drawn. 2.10(b) shows the results after using the same sequence of flows.

2.4.3 Testing

The algorithm was tested on real images of lamin and a6b1 integrin stained cells in culture and tissue to demonstrate the practical application of the approach. The images were selected to cover a range of situations of staining

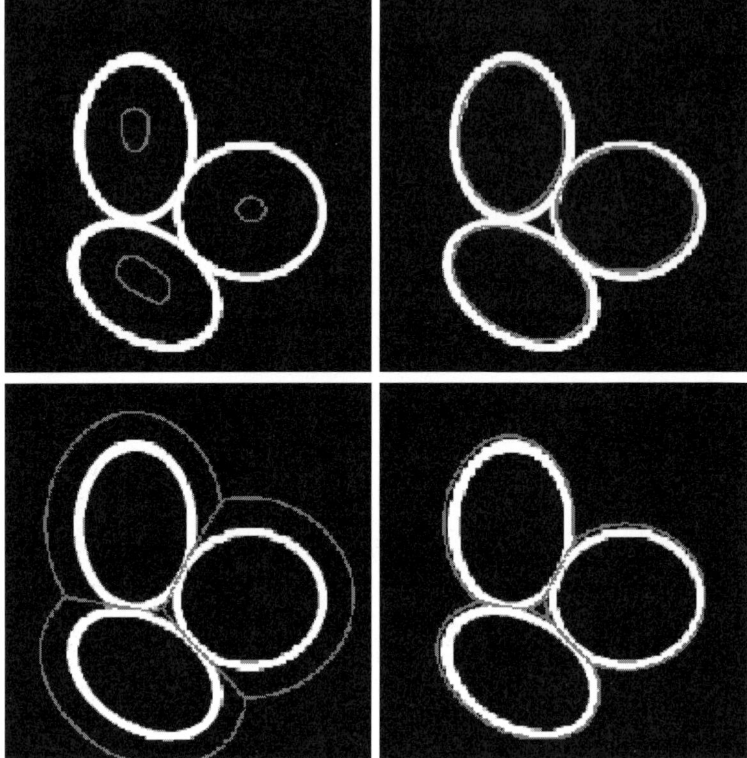

Fig. 2.9. Nuclear segmentation using a computer generated image (cont'd). (a) Top left: Surface of the seeds overimposed on the original image. (b) Top right: Initial expansion. (c) Bottom left: Free expansion. (d) Bottom right: Surface Wrapping.

quality and image noise which gave us confidence that the algorithm would work on images from a wide variety of specimens.

2.4.4   Results

All of the nuclei/cells that we used to test the algorithm were successfully segmented. We segmented 19 lamin stained nuclei from cultured cells, 24 a6b1 integrin stained cells from cultured cells and 23 a6b1 integrin stained cells in tissue.

Examples of the images, which are 2D images selected from the acquired confocal 3D sets (except 2D-conventional images of real tissue sections) are shown in Figures 2.11, 2.12 and 2.13, along with the results of the flow over imposed on the original images. Figure 2.11 shows two examples of the segmentation of nuclei in cultured cells stained with lamin antibodies. 2.12 shows two examples of whole cell segmentation using a6b1 integrin staining in cultured cells, where the cells formed acini mimicking ducts of the mammary

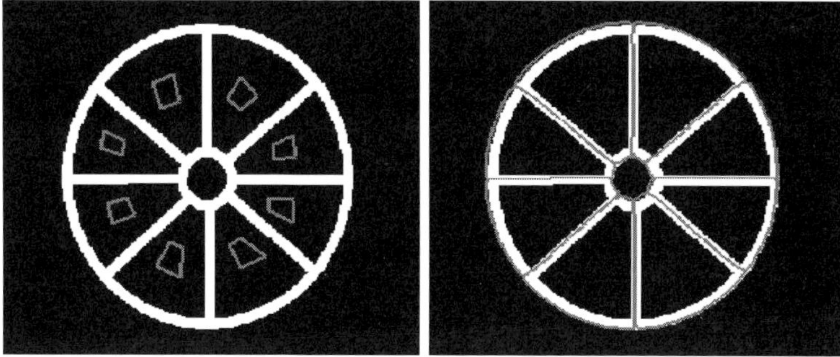

Fig. 2.10. Computer generated object simulating a group of epithelial a6b1 integrin stained cells. (a)Left: Manual initialization of the segmentation. (b)Right: Final segmentation result after applying the algorithm described in the text.

gland. Figure 2.13 shows whole cell segmentation in intact tissue stained with a6b1 integrin. Note that both figures 2.12 and 2.13 contain cells with concavities in their surfaces, which the algorithm was able to follow.

These examples demonstrate that the algorithm converges to the nuclear or cellular surface, and that it admits a range of variation in the quality of the staining within and between images. Some tuning of the parameters might be necessary to adapt the segmentation to images substantially different from the images used. The advantages of this approach are: it does not have strict initialization constraints in that the size, shape and position of the seed are not critical for providing an accurate segmentation; the flows can be adapted to local image characteristics, such as curvature, edge strength and direction, etc.; from the implementation point of view a discrete approach can be used to approximate the solution of the flow equation that describes the movement of the surface.

2.5 Conclusions

In this chapter we have presented some algorithms to solve diverse image analysis problems that one typically finds in the study of confocal microscope images.

These problems range from low-level feature-preserving noise elimination, nuclei or cell shape reconstruction, shape smoothing, certain morphological operations on the segmented shapes, hole removal, cluster elimination etc. Our approach was to use a unified geometric framework in which all of the aforementioned image analysis tasks are implemented efficiently as various interpretations of an underlying partial differential equation. We presented results on testing our method on real confocal microscope images.

Acknowledgments

This work was supported under Contract No. DE-AC03-76SF00098 of the

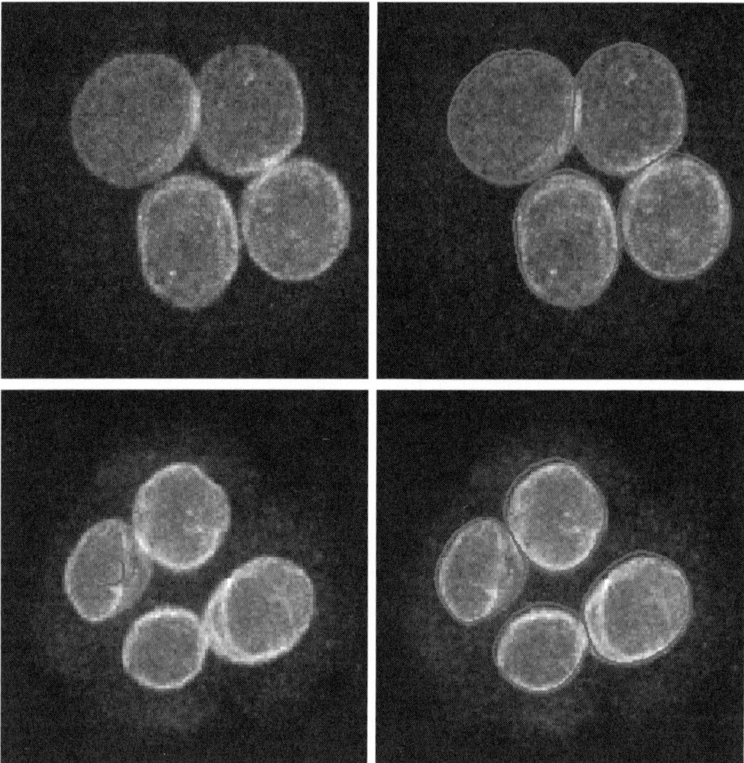

Fig. 2.11. Examples of the segmentation results on real images from cultured lamin stained cells. (a)and (c) Left column: Original images with the automatically detected seeds. (b) and (d)Right column: Results, overimposed on the original images.

U.S. Department of Energy's Office of Energy Research, Office of Computational and Technology Research, Mathematical, Information, and Computational Sciences Division, Applied Mathematical Sciences Subprogram; Director, Office of Energy Research, Office of Health and Environmental Research; ONR Grant under NOOO14-96-1-0381,and LBNL Directed Research and Development Program. This work was also supported by the U.S. National Institutes of Health Grant CA-67412, a contract with Zeiss Inc., and by the Training program in Genome Research of the UC Systemwide Biotechnology Research and Education Program.

References

1. Adalsteinsson D. and Sethian J.A.: A fast level set method for propagating interfaces. J. Comp. Phys. bf 118(2) (1995) 269–277
2. Alvarez L., Guichard F., Lions P. L., and Morel J. M.: Axioms and fundamental equations of image processing. Arch. Rational Mechanics **123** (1993)

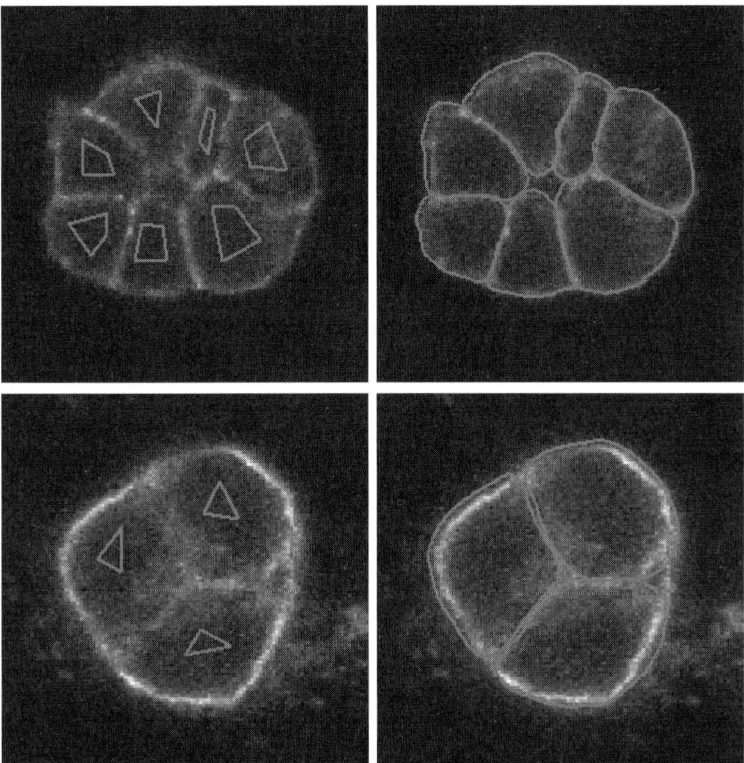

Fig. 2.12. Examples of the segmentation results on cultured a6b1 integrin stained cells. (a) and (c) Left column: Original images with the interactively detected seeds. (b) and (d) Right column: Results, overimposed on the original images. The white arrows in figure (b) show concavities that were followed by the algorithm.

3. Ancin H , Roysam R.,Dufresne T.E., Chesnut M.M., Ridder G.M., Szarowski D.H., TurnerJ.N.: Advances in Automated 3-D Image Analysis of Cell Populations Imaged by Confocal Microscopy. Cytometry **25** (1996) 221–234

4. Ballard DH.: Generalizing the Hough Transform to detect arbitrary shapes. Pattern Recogn. **13** (1981) 111–122.

5. Balzer P., Furber A., Cavaro-Menard C., Croue A., Tadei A., Geslin P., Jallet P., Le Jeune JJ.: Simultaneous and correlated detection of endocardial and epicardial borders on short-axis MR images for the measurement of left ventricular mass. Radiographics **18** (1998) 1009–1018.

6. Bart M., Haar Romeny(Ed.): Geometry-driven diffusion in computer vision. Kluwer Academic Press, 1994

7. Bosman F.T.: Integrins: cell adhesives and modulators of cell function. Histochem. J. **25** (1993) 469-477

8. Caselles V., Catte F., Coll T., Dibos F.: A geometric model for active contours. Numerische Mathematik **66** (1993) 1–31

9. Caselles V., Kimmel R., Sapiro G.: Geodesic active contours. in Proc. ICCV'95, Cambridge, MA 1995

10. Cohen LD., Cohen I.: Finite-element methods for active contour models and balloons for 2-D and 3-D images. IEEE T. Pattern Anal. **15** (1993) 1131–1146.

11. Czader M., Liljeborg A., Auer G., Porwit A.: Confocal 3-Dimensional DNA Image Cytometry in Thick Tissue Sections. Cytometry **25** (1996) 246–253

12. Dastidar P., Heinonen T., Numminen J., Rautiainen M., Laasonen E.: Semi-automatic segmentation of computed tomographic images in volumetric estimation of nasal airway. Eur. Arch. Oto-rhino-l. **256** (1999) 192–198.

13. Dean P., Mascio L., Ow D., Sudar D., Mullikin J.: Proposed standard for image cytometry data files. Cytometry **11** (1990) 561–569

14. Grayson M.: The heat equation shrinks embedded plane curves to round points. J. Differential Geometry **26** (1987) 285–314

15. Heppner G. H.: Cell-to-cell interaction in regulating diversity of neoplasms. Seminars in Cancer Biology **2** (1991) 97–103

16. Irinopoulou T., Vassy J., Beil M., Nicolopoulou P., Encaoua D., Rigaut J.P.: Three-Dimensional DNA Image Cytometry by Confocal Scanning Laser Microscopy in Thick Tissue Blocks of Prostatic Lesions. Cytometry **27** (1997) 99–105

17. Kikinis R., Guttman CRG., Metcalf MS., Wells WM., Gil J., Ettinger MD., Howard L., Weiner MD., Jolesz FA.: Quantitative follow-up of patients with multiple sclerosis using MRI: Technical aspects. J. Magn. Reson. Imaging **9** (1999) 519–530

18. Koukoulis G.K., Virtanen I., Korhonen M., Laitinen L. Quarana V., Gould V.E.: Immunohistochemical localization of integrins in the normal, hyperplastic and neoplastic breast. Am. J. Pathol. bf 139 (1991) 787–799

19. Lelievre S., Weaver V.M., Bissell M.J.: Extracellular matrix signaling from the cellular membrane skeleton to the nuclear skeleton: A model of gene regulation. Recent Progress in Hormone Research **51** (1996) 417–432

20. Lockett S.J., Sudar D., Thompson C.T., Pinkel D., Gray J.W.: Efficient, interactive, three-dimensional segmentation of cell nuclei in thick tissue sections. Cytometry **31** (1998) 275–286

21. Malladi R., Sethian J.A., Vemuri B.C.: A topology-independent shape modeling scheme. in SPIE: Geometric Methods in Computer Vision II, Vol. 2031 (1993) 246–258

22. Malladi R., Sethian J.A., Vemuri B.C.: Shape modeling with front propagation: A level set approach. IEEE Trans. on PAMI **17** (1995) 158–175

23. Malladi R., Sethian J.A.: Image processing: Flows under Min/Max curvature and mean curvature. Graphical Models and Image Processing **58** (1996) 127–141

24. Malladi R., Sethian J.A.: Level set methods for curvature flow, image enchancement and shape recovery in medical images. in Visualization and Mathematics: Experiments, Simulations, and Environments, Eds. H. C. Hege, K. Polthier, pp. 329–345, Springer Verlag, Heidelberg, 1997.

25. Malladi R., Sethian J.A.: A real-time algorithm for medical shape recovery. in Proceedings of ICCV '98, pp. 304–310, Mumbai India, January 1998.

26. Mikula K., Sarti A., Lamberti C.: Geometrical diffusion in 3D echocardiography. Proc. of ALGORITMY '97- Conference on Scientific Computing, West Tatra Mountains, Slovakia, 1997.

27. Miller F.R., Heppner G.H.: Cellular interactions in metastasis. Cancer and Metastasis Reviews **9** (1990) 21–34
28. Mullikin J.C.: The vector distance transform in two and three dimensions. CVGIP: Graphical Models and Image Processing **54** (1992) 526–535
29. Nordstrom N.K.: Variational edge detection. PhD dissertation, Department of electrical engineering, University of California, Berkeley, 1990
30. Ortiz de Solorzano C., Garcia Rodriguez E., Jones A., Pinkel D., Gray J.W., Sudar D., Lockett S.J.: Segmentation of confocal microscope images of cell nuclei in thick tissue sections. Journal of Microscopy **193** (1999) 212–226
31. Ortiz de Solorzano C., Malladi R., Lelievre S., Lockett S.J.: Segmentation of Cell and Nuclei using Membrane Related Proteins. Journal of Microscopy-Oxford **201** (2001) 1–13
32. Osher S.J., Sethian J.A.: Fronts propagation with curvature dependent speed: Algorithms based on Hamilton-Jacobi formulations. Journal of Computational Physics **79** (1988) 12–49
33. Rigaut J.P., Vassy J., Herlin P., Duigou F., Masson E., Briane D., Foucrier J., Carvajal-Gonzalez S., Downs A.M., Mandard A-M.: Three-Dimensional DNA Image Cytometry by Confocal Scanning Laser Microscopy in Thick Tissue Blocks. Cytometry **12** (1991) 511–524
34. Sapiro G.: Color snakes. Hewlett-Packard Lab. tech report, 1995
35. Sapiro G., Kimmel R., Shaked D., Kimia B.B., Bruckstein A.M.: Implementing continuous-scale morphology via curve evolution. Pattern Recognition **6** (1993) 1363–1372
36. Sarti A., Mikula K., Sgallari F.: Nonlinear multiscale analysis of 3D echocardiographic sequences IEEE Trans. on Medical Imaging **18** (1999) 453–466
37. Sarti A., Ortiz de Solorzano C., Lockett S., Malladi R.: A Geometric Model for 3-D Confocal Image Analysis IEEE Trans. on Biomedical Engineering **47** (2000) 1600-1609
38. Sethian J.A.: A review of recent numerical algorithms for hypersurfaces moving with curvature dependent flows. J. Differential Geometry **31** (1989) 131–161
39. Sethian J.A.: Level set methods: Evolving interfaces in geometry, fluid mechanics, computer vision, and material science. Cambridge University Press, 1997
40. Sochen N., Kimmel R., Malladi R.: A General Framework for Low Level Vision. IEEE Transactions on Image Processing, special issue on PDEs and Geometry-Driven Diffusion in Image Processing and Analysis **7** (1998) 310–318
41. Wilson T.: Confocal Microscopy, Academic Press, London, 1990.

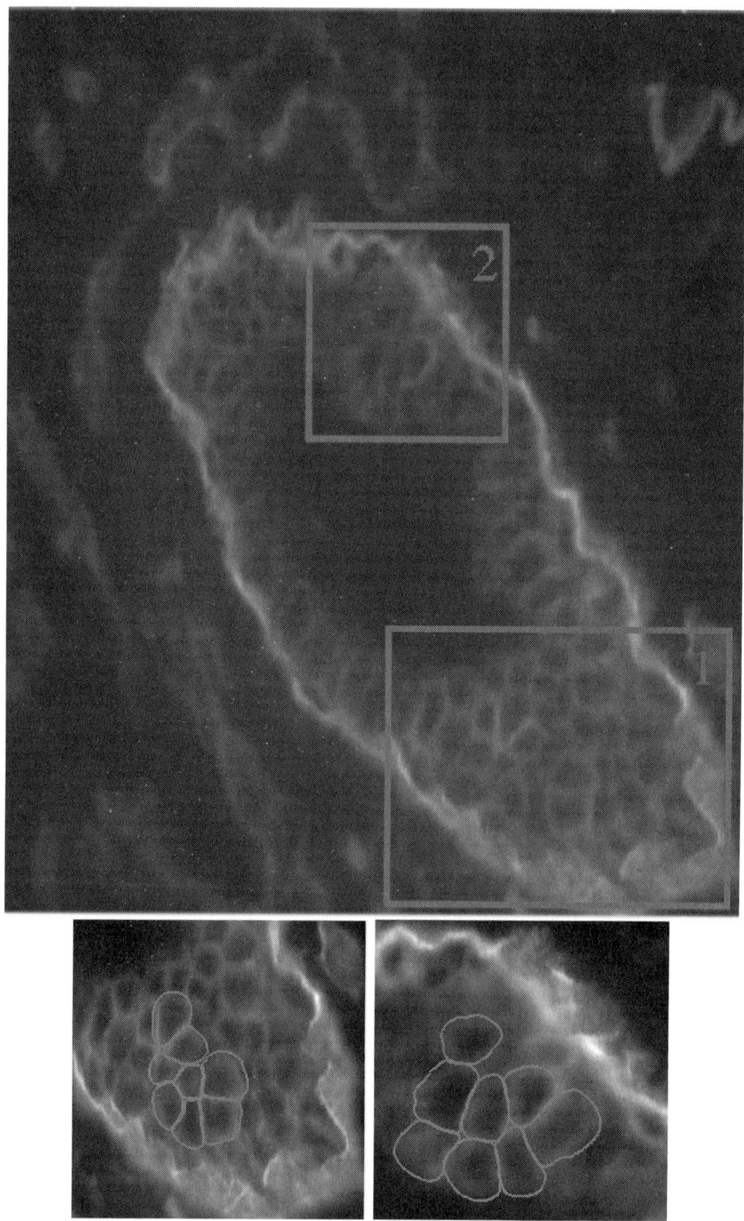

Fig. 2.13. Example of the segmentation results on two parts (b) and (c) of a mouse mammary tissue stained for a6b1 integrin. (a) Top: Original image. (b) and (c) Bottom: show Results on interactively seeded nuclei from two parts of image a.

3 Level Set Models for Analysis of $2D$ and $3D$ Echocardiographic Data

A. Sarti[2], C. Lamberti[2], and R. Malladi[1]

[1] Department of Mathematics, University of California, Berkeley and Lawrence Berkeley National Laboratory, University of California,Berkeley, USA
[2] DEIS, University of Bologna, Italy

Abstract. We propose a partial differential equation (PDE) for filtering and segmentation of echocardiographic images based on a geometric-driven scheme. The method allows edge-preserving image smoothing and a semi-automatic segmentation of the heart chambers, that regularizes the shapes and improves edge fidelity especially in presence of distinct gaps in the edge map as is common in ultrasound imagery. A numerical scheme for solving the proposed PDE is borrowed from level set methods. Results on human in vivo acquired 2D, 2D+time,3D, 3D+time echocardiographic images are shown.

3.1 Introduction

Heart muscle failure is one of the primary cause of death among human beings. Therefore, evaluation of heart function is an important component in good health care. Echocardiography is by far the most commonly used imaging technique to diagnose pathologies of the cardiac muscle. The features that have made it so largely used are its noninvasiveness, ease of use, low cost and effectiveness in diagnosing heart pathologies. $2D$ echocardiography only allows visualization of planar tomographic sections of the heart; thus, it relies on strong geometrical assumptions for the determination of heart chamber volume and it is subject to considerable measurement error, especially for the right ventricular and atrial volume determination [3]. On the other hand, $3D$ echocardiography overcomes the need for geometrical assumptions, thereby allowing accurate evaluation of chambers size and shape, even in case of cavities with irregular geometry.

A serious drawback is the poor quality of echograms if compared, for example, with Computed Tomography (CT) or Magnetic Resonance (MR). An accurate visualization and interpretation of ultrasounds images is often affected by the high amount of noise intrinsically linked to the acquisition method. Indeed the process of formation of an ultrasound image involves a combination of coherent, rayleigh and diffractive scattering that produces the characteristic speckle-noise distribution [35]. Traditional pre-processing algorithms such as moving average, median and Gaussian filtering reduce the noise superimposed on the image but do not preserve the edge information or the boundaries [10]. Non-linear filtering methods based on partial differential equations have been applied in [18,9,26].

Many techniques have been proposed in the literature to extract the ventricular surface in conditions of end-systole and end-diastole – thus when the ventricle is closed – starting from a small number of $2D$ images that represent different sections of the ventricle. Reconstruction of the ventricular chamber has been widely studied in recent years from Computed Tomography and Magnetic Resonance Imaging. Cohen in [6][7] uses the concept of active deformable contours for the segmentation of ventricular shapes from $2D$ echocardiography and $3D$ magnetic resonance. The approach is a generalization of Kass, Witkin, and Terzopoulos deformable elastic model [12]. Malladi, Sethian, and Vemuri in [13,14] combine the idea of deformable surfaces with the level-set approach of Osher and Sethian [20], by representing the surface as a particular level-set of an implicit function and applying it to the reconstruction of the ventricular chamber in $3D+$ time MR images; see [16].

The difficulty in segmenting the heart chamber shapes from echocardiograms is two fold; first, the images are relatively noisy resulting in poor edge indicator and second, due to opening and closing of the heart valve, the boundary of the left ventricle remains uncertain in some images. Big 'holes' due to open valves many times causes the shape model to erroneously flow into the atrium. We address both these issues in this paper. The noise and poor edge quality is handled with an edge preserving filtering mechanism [36] and the issue of shape uncertainty is resolved by exploiting the continuity assumption in time [26].

In this paper we want to address both the tasks of edge preserving image denoising and shape extraction of the cardiac chambers from echocardiographic images, by using the same geometric partial differential equation (PDE) based model. Encouraged by the recent advances [14][15] [16]-[17][36][2][23] [26][28] [29][30][18] in PDE based image analysis tools, we extend and apply some of those methods to echocardiographic image analysis. The theme of this paper is to start with a governing equation that is expressed via an Euler-Lagrange of a functional and to show its many interpretations. A numerical scheme based on the level set methods [20] and the efficient narrow-band versions [1][14] of it are used to solve the main equation.

Another key aspect of this paper is the accurate estimation of ventricular volume from the extracted shapes. This leads to the estimation of such quantities as ejection fraction from a time varying set of $3D$ images. Finally, to demonstrate the accuracy of our segmentation scheme, we compare the volume figures we obtain from segmenting sheep heart images to the exact experimentally measured values [21,22].

The rest of the paper is organized as follows: In Section 2 we present the main equation and we outline its relevant features. In Section 3 we interpret the main equation as an image processing algorithm and show its application in echocardiographic image denoising. In Section 4 we study the geometric interpretation of the model for shape segmentation. In Section 5-8 results of the application of the model to in vivo ultrasound acquisitions are presented and details of the implementation are provided.

3.2   The Geometric Evolution Equation

Consider an hypersurface $\Upsilon(x, t)$ that is propagating under the speed $\mathcal{F}$ in the normal direction. The speed $\mathcal{F}(N, \mathcal{K}, x)$ is a function of the intrinsic geometrical properties of the hypersurface, like the normal vector and curvature, as well as of the position. We consider a level set equation [20][32][33] to represent this motion by embedding the hypersurface as the zero level-set of an higher dimensional function $\Psi(x, t)$, namely the set $\{\Psi(x, t) = 0\}$. By following chain rule, the equation of motion of the embedding is

$$\Psi_t + \mathcal{F}|\nabla\Psi| = 0 \tag{3.1}$$

with the initial condition $\Psi(x, t = 0) = \Psi_0$. By embedding the evolution of $\Upsilon(x, t)$ in the evolution of $\Psi(x, t)$, topological changes of $\Upsilon(x, t)$ are handled automatically and a numerical solution for the evolutionary hypersurface can be accurately achieved in the viscosity framework presented in [20]. Several applications in shape modeling have been presented using this model for surface propagation in [13][4][14][16]. Level set methods in image analysis have been introduced in [14] for boundary extraction. The method relies on evolving an initial manifold in the image domain and to mold the shape into the desired boundary. The key is a suitable design of the evolution speed $\mathcal{F}$. In [14] the speed function used to control the shape recovery process is a combination of constant inflationary speed, an intrinsic geometric speed that regularizes the final result and a speed that depends on the image:

$$\mathcal{F} = g\left(1 - \epsilon\nabla \cdot \frac{\nabla\Psi}{|\nabla\Psi|}\right) \tag{3.2}$$

where g is a decreasing function of the image gradient. It has to be noted that the curvature of the hypersurface written as a function of the level set of $\Psi(x, t)$ is just $\mathcal{K} = \nabla \cdot \frac{\nabla\Psi}{|\nabla\Psi|}$ and then the above expression defines the propagation of $\Upsilon(x, t)$ driven by the image features and regularized by the curvature; $\mathcal{K}$ is the Euclidean curvature for plane curves and the mean curvature for manifolds.

In addition to the speed term in Eqn. 3.2, an attraction to the boundary features can be defined by adding a forcing term that advects the surface along an image dependent vector field [5][16]. The vector field has to be synthesized such that it always points towards the local edge. The speed function then takes the form:

$$\mathcal{F} = g\left(1 - c\mathcal{K}\right) - \beta\nabla g \cdot \left(\frac{\nabla\Psi}{|\nabla\Psi|}\right), \tag{3.3}$$

where the unit normal to the surface is expressed by the term $N = -\frac{\nabla\Psi}{|\nabla\Psi|}$. The corresponding surface evolution has a steady state solution when the inflationary and the geometry dependent terms balance the advection term. As shown in [5,16], this model of surface evolution leads to stable shape recovery even in the presence of minor gaps and oscillations along the edge. However, echocardiographic images are significantly noisier with much poorer edge definition when compared to CT, and MR images. They not only have noisy structures but often large parts of the boundaries are missing making the shape recovery really troublesome. So, even with the extra forcing term in Eqn. 3.3, the evolving "edge-seeking" surface can easily go through the gaps present in the edge map. We aim to develop a filtering and segmentation method that deals with non-continuous edges.

We propose the following evolution equation for the level set function Ψ:

$$\Psi_t - g\mathcal{K}|\nabla\Psi| - \beta\nabla g \cdot \nabla\Psi = 0. \qquad (3.4)$$

Notice that the constant component of the speed, i.e. the 'edge-seeking" term has been dropped. The reason for this change is two fold: (a) given a good initial condition, the segmentation algorithm will recover shapes with significant gaps by simply minimizing distance in areas where edge information is absent, and (2) as we show in the next section, the above equation can be used to denoise the original image as well as enhance edges. The edge enhancement step is used as a precursor to segmentation. The equation itself can be solved with user-defined initial condition during the segmentation step and with the original image as an initial condition for the edge-enhancement stage. The model regularizes the boundaries where a clear representation of the edges is missed. It presents topological adaptability, robust numerics and very fast implementations [17].

3.3   The Shock-Type Filtering

Low level image processing tends to achieve the basic result of computing a decomposition $\{\Omega_i\}$ of the domain $\Omega = \Omega_1 \cup \ldots \cup \Omega_N$ and computing an enhanced image similar to the original one, that varies smoothly and slowly within each Ω_i and discontinuously on (part of) the boundary of the Ω_i. Boundaries of the homogeneous regions Ω_i that are not part of the boundary of Ω are called edges[1]. The goal is then to smooth all the homogeneous regions that contain noise and to retain in an accurate way the location of the edges that define the shape of the represented structures. We shall now show how we can use Eqn 3.4 to do image processing. Let us consider an image $I_0(x) : \Omega \rightarrow$, where $\Omega \subset R^N$ is a rectangular spatial domain and $N = 2$ for $2D$ images and $N = 3$ for $3D$ images. The image filtering associates with $I_0(x)$ a family $\Psi(x, t) : \Omega \times [0, T] \rightarrow R$ of simplified-filtered images depending on an abstract parameter t, the *scale*. To better understand the method, let us consider the main equation, namely:

$$\Psi_t = g\left(\nabla \cdot \frac{\nabla\Psi}{|\nabla\Psi|}\right)|\nabla\Psi| + \beta\nabla g \cdot \nabla\Psi$$

$$g(x) = \frac{1}{1 + (|\nabla G_\sigma(x) \star I_0(x)|/\alpha)^2}$$

$$G_\sigma(\xi) = \frac{\exp(-(\xi/\sigma)^2)}{\sigma\sqrt{\pi}} \tag{3.5}$$

with the initial condition given by the noisy image $\Psi(x, t = 0) = I_0(x)$.

The first (parabolic) term in Eqn. 3.5 is a geometric diffusion term weighted by the edge indicator g. The geometric diffusion term $\left(\nabla \cdot \frac{\nabla\Psi}{|\nabla\Psi|}\right)|\nabla\Psi|$ is a degenerate diffusion term that diffuses the signal only in the direction parallel to the boundaries and not at all in the direction of $\nabla\Psi$ thereby preserving edge definition. Writing the diffusion term as Morel and Solimini noted that:

$$\left(\nabla \cdot \frac{\nabla\Psi}{|\nabla\Psi|}\right)|\nabla\Psi| = \Delta\Psi - \frac{D^2(\nabla\Psi, \nabla\Psi)}{|\nabla\Psi|^2} \tag{3.6}$$

Morel and Solimini noted that the first term, the Laplacian, is the same as in Scale Space Theory [2] and the second one is an inhibition of the diffusion in the direction of the gradient. The weighting function g enforces edge preservation by slowing down the geometric diffusion in presence of high gradient in the smoothed image. Thus the aim of the selective geometric diffusion term is to make Ψ smooth away from the edges with a minimal smoothing of the edge itself. The second (hyperbolic) term in Eqn 3.5 sharpens the edges by advecting the brightness signal of the initial image I_0 toward the edges following the vector fields induced by ∇g. A similar observation was made in [24].

The edge indicator $g(x)$ is a non-increasing function of $\nabla G_\sigma(x) \star I_0(x)$. To interpret this term we observe that the convolution property $\nabla G_\sigma(x) \star I_0(x) - \nabla(G_\sigma(x) \star I_0(x)) - G_\sigma(x) \star \nabla I_0(x)$ holds. Thus we can consider it as the gradient of a smoothed version of the initial image: $I_s(x) = G_\sigma(x) \star I_0(x)$. We compute it via heat-flow (an idea usually attributed to Koendrink) by observing that the convolution of the signal with Gaussian is equivalent to the solution of the heat equation:

$$I_s(x, t) = \int_0^\sigma \Delta I(x, t)dt \tag{3.7}$$

$$I(x, 0) = I_0(x).$$

In the filtering process the minimal size of the details that are preserved is related to the size of the Gauss kernel, which acts like a scale parameter. Notice that the filtering model reduces to mean curvature flow when $g(s) = 1$.

We have applied the multiscale analysis model to an in vivo acquired 2D and 3D echocardiographic sequence. The sequence has been obtained by means of a rotational acquisition technique using the TomTec Imaging System. With this technique the transducer undergoes a rotation around its main axis in a propeller configuration. A series of tomographies corresponding to the sections of a cone of biological tissue have been acquired. The acquisition consists of 14 image-cubes that represent a whole cardiac cycle of a real patient. A volume of size 151 x 151 x 101 voxels has been processed. The interval of time between one $3D$ image and the next one is 40 ms.

In Figure 3.1 a slice of the $3D$ volume has been visualized. The original noisy image is shown on the left and the result of the multiscale denoising algorithm with $\alpha = 0.1, \beta = 1.5, \Delta t = 0.05$, and $\sigma = 0.001$ is presented on the right. In Figures 3.2–3.5 a sequence of filtered volumes is shown. The parameters are the same as in the $2D$ computation. The iso-surfaces corresponding to the interface between cardiac muscle and blood have been computed using the marching cubes method and visualized by a Gouraud surface rendering ([11], [34]). To clarify the visualization of the ventricular chambers we applied four cutting planes that isolate the region of interest. In clinical practice a cutting plane that filters out the "front" regions is often used. The epicardium is not visible because the gray levels of his interface are not captured by the marching cubes threshold we have chosen in order to visualize the left ventricle. In particular the low echogenicity of the blood allows the choice of a low isosurface threshold that avoids the visualization of most of the other structures.

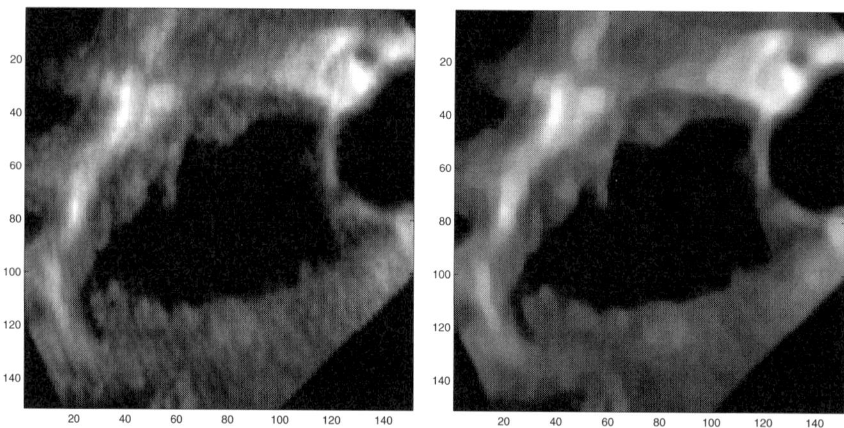

Fig. 3.1. $2D$ echocardiography of in vivo acquired left ventricle. Left: original image. Right: result of geometric image denoising.

Note that the $3D$ pictures are simply meant to visually demonstrate the degree of noise reduction via the proposed geometric method. A more thorough study involving measuring the degree of noise reduction and a detailed comparison with other denoising schemes has been done in another work [27].

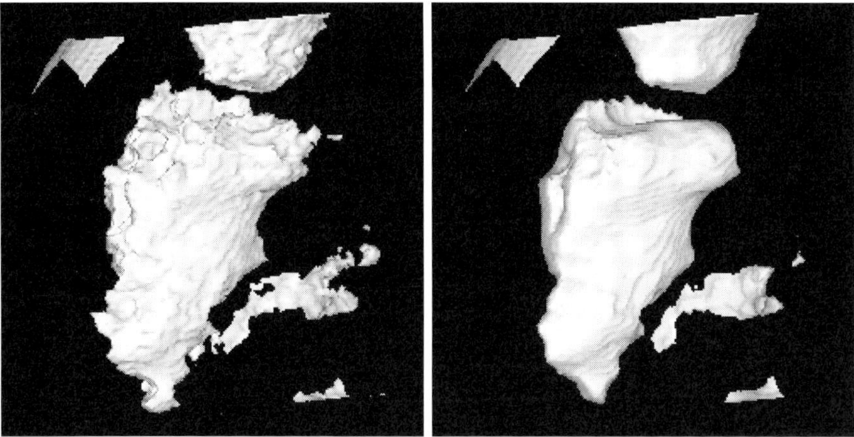

Fig. 3.2. Geometric smoothing of the 1st frame of the 3D echocardiographic sequence.

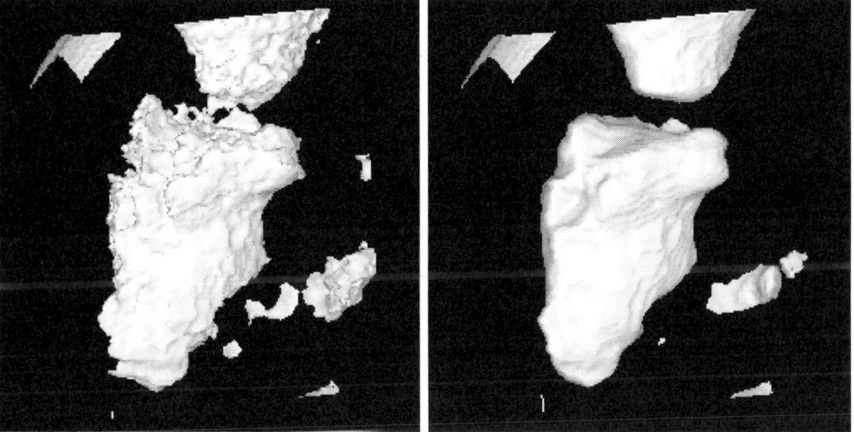

Fig. 3.3. Geometric smoothing of the 5th frame of the 3D echocardiographic sequence.

The rendered surfaces cannot be used for any measurement or tracking. The problem of explicitly building a shape model of the shape of interest is the topic of next section.

3.4   Shape Extraction

Imagine a planar curve C_0 in an image $I(x) : \Omega \rightarrow R^+, \Omega \subset R^N, N = 2,$ and consider the evolution $C(t)$ of that initial shape. We want to study the evolution rules that allows us to mold the curve conformally into the edge

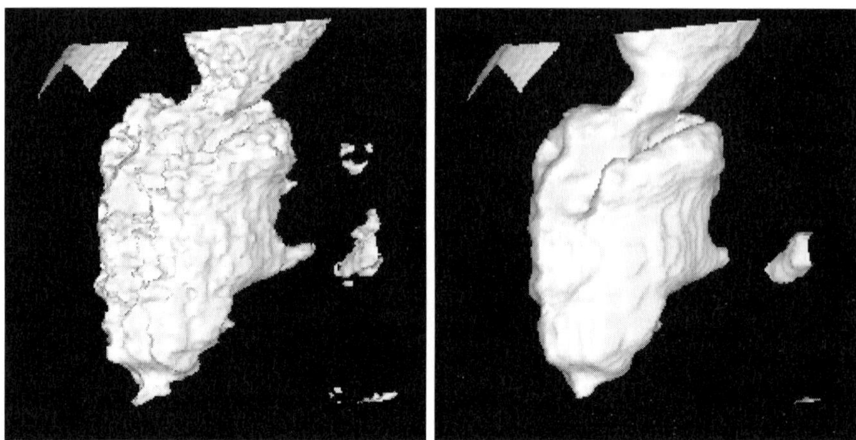

Fig. 3.4. Geometric smoothing of the 9th frame of the 3D echocardiographic sequence.

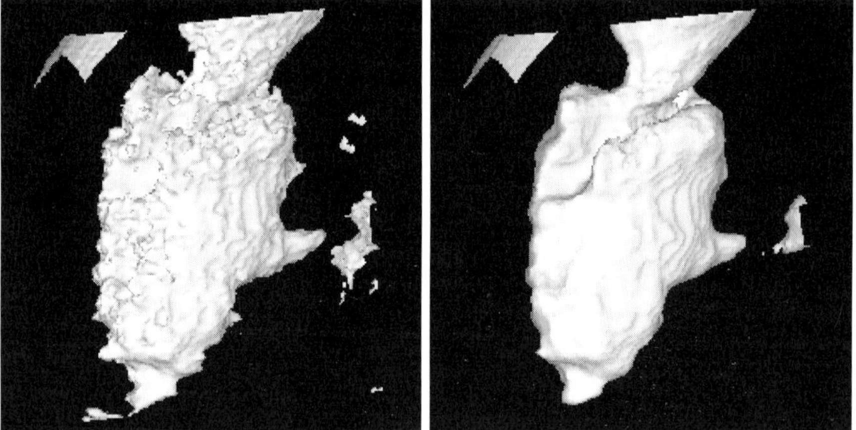

Fig. 3.5. Geometric smoothing of the 13th frame of the 3D echocardiographic sequence.

map. Consider first the basic motion:

$$C_t = F\mathbf{N} \tag{3.8}$$

where $\mathbf{N}$ is the unit inward normal and F is a real function. The curve moves with speed F in the normal direction. Let us design F in such a way that $C(t)$ is attracted by the boundaries in the image. Consider the following evolution equation:

$$C_t = (-\nabla g \cdot \mathbf{N})\mathbf{N}. \tag{3.9}$$

Recall that the minima of the edge indicator $g(x)$ denote the position of the edges and therefore the vector field $-\nabla g$ can be shown to point toward the edges. The result of this flow is an oscillatory curve without "smoothness" or regularization.

One way of introducing smoothness in the curve is to let it evolve under its Euclidean curvature K,

$$C_t = K\mathbf{N}. \tag{3.10}$$

This flow decreases the Euclidean curvature and has the property of smoothing all the high curvature regions of the curve, i.e. the local variations [8]. However, this flow will also destroy useful curve features if run long enough. Thus a key point is to determine a suitable stopping criterion. Several methods have been proposed in the past in the framework of variational methods [19] and level set methods [15]. The authors in [15] have presented a scale-dependent stopping criteria implemented via a min-max curvature flow. In the present context we use the function g to introduce the stopping criterion. Therefore the evolution equation for curve regularization becomes:

$$C_t = gK\mathbf{N} \tag{3.11}$$

where the curvature motion is slowed down near the shape boundaries. The final evolution equation for shape extraction will use both the attraction and the regularization terms, namely

$$C_t = (gK - \beta(\nabla g \cdot \mathbf{N}))\mathbf{N} \tag{3.12}$$

where the initial condition $C(0) = C_0$ is any curve sufficiently close to the boundary to feel the effect of the edge map $g(x)$.

In [16,17], the above curve evolution model has been extended to surface evolution for segmentation of 3D shapes from volumetric images. In this case we define a surface S_0 in an image $I(x) : \Omega \rightarrow R^+, \Omega \subset R^N, N = 3$ and evolve the surface towards the shape boundaries. Applying an analogous argument will lead us to write the following surface evolution equation for 3D segmentation:

$$S_t = (gH - \beta(\nabla g \cdot \mathbf{N}))\mathbf{N}, \tag{3.13}$$

where H is the mean curvature and $\mathbf{N}$ is the normal to the surface.

The curve and surface evolution in Eqns. 3.12 and 3.13 can be solved using the level-set approach [20][33] . Consider an $(N-1)$-dimensional hypersurface $\Upsilon(x,t)$ ($N = 2$ for C and $N = 3$ for S) and represent it as the zero level-set of a function $\Psi(x,t) : \Omega \times [0,T] \rightarrow R, \Omega \subset R^N, N = 2,3$. In other words, the initial curve or surface is simply the set $\{\Psi = 0\}$. The function Ψ therefore is an implicit representation of the hypersurface. Both Eqns. 3.12 and 3.13 have the same level-set form, i.e. the main model:

$$\Psi_t = g\left(\nabla \cdot \frac{\nabla\Psi}{|\nabla\Psi|}\right)|\nabla\Psi| + \beta\nabla g \cdot \nabla\Psi$$

$$g(x) = \frac{1}{1 + (|\nabla I_{GS}(x)|/\alpha)^2} \tag{3.14}$$

with the initial condition $\Psi(x, t = 0) = \Psi_0$. In our case Ψ_0 is the signed distance function from the initial hypersurface $\Upsilon(x, t = 0)$. Note that the function g is an edge indicator expressed as a non-increasing function of the image gradient. The gradient is computed from a geometrically enhanced image, denoted as I_{GS}, using Eqn. 3.4. This also establishes a link between the two stages of processing we employ in this work. In the next section we show how the image analysis methodology developed in the last two sections can be utilized to build accurate shape descriptions from echocardiograms.

3.5 $2D$ Echocardiography

Consider a 2D echocardiographic image $I(x)$ from which we want to accurately extract the boundaries of the cardiac chamber. We consider the embedding $\varphi : \Omega \times [0, T] \to R, \Omega \subset R^2$ and look for the steady state of the evolution equation:

$$\varphi_t = gK|\nabla\varphi| + \beta\nabla g \cdot \nabla\varphi \tag{3.15}$$

$$g(x) = \frac{1}{1 + (|\nabla I_{GS}(x)|/\alpha)^2} \tag{3.16}$$

with the initial condition given by a user-defined signed distance function $\varphi(x, 0) = \varphi_0$. The Euclidean curvature K is obtained from the divergence of the unit normal vector:

$$K = \frac{\varphi_{xx}\varphi_y^2 - 2\varphi_x\varphi_y\varphi_{xy} + \varphi_{yy}\varphi_x^2}{(\varphi_x^2 + \varphi_y^2)^{3/2}}. \tag{3.17}$$

We now show how to approximate the above equation with finite differences. Let us consider a rectangular uniform grid in space-time (t, x, y); then the grid will be the points $(t_n, x_i, y_j) = (n\Delta t, i\Delta x, j\Delta y)$. We use the notation φ_{ij}^n for the value of φ at the grid point (t_n, x_i, y_j). The curvature term is a parabolic contribution to the equation of motion. In terms of numerical scheme we approximate this with central differences. The second term on the right corresponds to pure passive advection by the underlying velocity field ∇g whose direction and strength depend on position. This term can be approximated through upwind schemes for hyperbolic terms, as noted in [33]. In other words, we check the sign of each component of ∇g and construct one-sided upwind differences in the appropriate direction. We can write now the complete first order scheme to approximate the above equation as

$$\varphi_{ij}^{n+1} = \varphi_{ij}^n + \Delta t \left[\begin{array}{c} [g_{ij}K_{ij}^n(D_{ij}^{0x^2} + D_{ij}^{0y^2})^{1/2}] \\ - \left\{ \begin{array}{l} [max(g_{ij}^{0x}, 0)D_{ij}^{-x} + min(g_{ij}^{0x}, 0)D_{ij}^{+x} \\ +max(g_{ij}^{0y}, 0)D_{ij}^{-y} + min(g_{ij}^{0y}, 0)D_{ij}^{+y}] \end{array} \right\} \end{array} \right] \tag{3.18}$$

where D is a finite difference operator on φ, the superscripts $\{-, 0, +\}$ indicate backward, central and forward differences respectively, and the superscripts

$\{x, y\}$ indicate the direction of differentiation. In Figures 3.6-3.7, we show the steps involved in the extraction of the heart chamber shape from a noisy echocardiogram. Figure 3.8 shows the result of ventricular chamber extraction from another echocardiogram data set. Here we make two observations, (1) the algorithm faithfully reconstructs the shape of the heart chamber inspite of large gaps in the edge map, and (2) the algorithm requires the user to place the initial contour reasonably close to the final shape as opposed to mere shape tagging approach described in [17]. This is because we have eliminated the constant inflationary or "edge-seeking" term (Eqn. 3.2) that was used in [14] to prevent the contour model from propagating past the edge gaps. So, in areas of image with little or no edge information, the length-minimizing curvature term takes over and closes the gap.

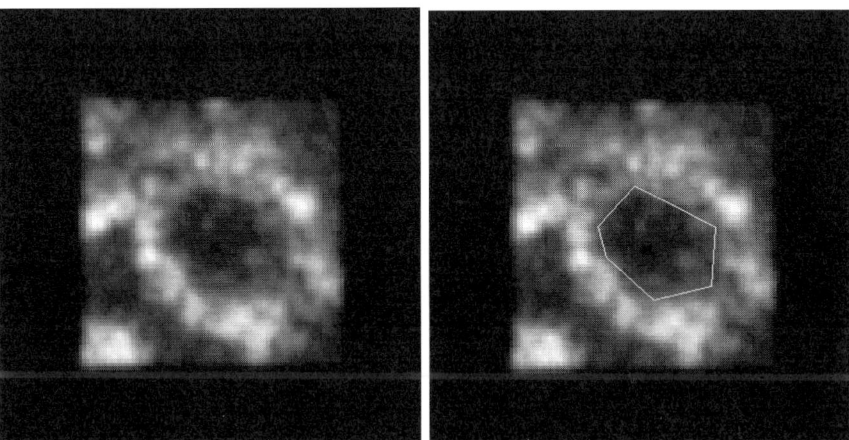

Fig. 3.6. Extraction of the ventricular chamber from a $2D$ echocardiogram. Left: Initial noisy image with many gaps in the edge description. Right: User defined initial contour expressed as the zero level-set of a function.

3.6 $2D + time$ Echocardiography

The requirement of placing the initial contour reasonably close to the final solution is both restrictive and time consuming. In this section, we address the issue of analyzing a time varying sequence of echocardiographic images. Let us now consider a time sequence of $2D$ echocardiographic images that represents an entire cardiac cycle $I^{(m)}, m = 1 \ldots M$. We segment the cardiac chamber by extending the geometric model to the time sequence, as follows:

$$\varphi_t^{(m)} = g^{(m)} K^{(m)} |\nabla \varphi^{(m)}| + \beta \nabla g^{(m)} \cdot \nabla \varphi^{(m)} \tag{3.19}$$

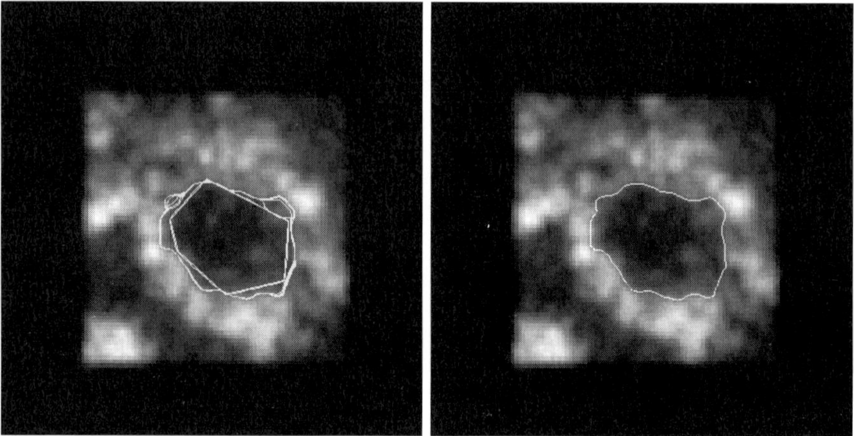

Fig. 3.7. Extraction of the ventricular chamber from a $2D$ echocardiogram. Left: Various stages of evolutions rendered on the same image, Right: Steady state solution of the level set evolution.

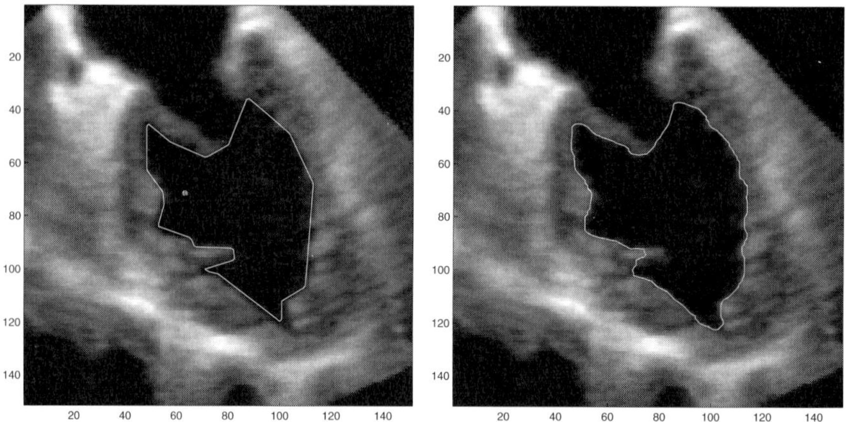

Fig. 3.8. Extraction of the ventricular chamber from a $2D$ echocardiogram. Left: zero level set of the signed distance function used as initial condition Right: Steady state solution of the level set evolution.

$$g^{(m)}(x) = \frac{1}{1 + (|\nabla I_{GS}^{(m)}(x)|/\alpha)^2} \qquad (3.20)$$

where the initial conditions are $\varphi_0^{(0)} = \varphi_0$ and $\varphi_0^{(m)} = \varphi_{ss}^{(m-1)}, m = 1 \ldots M$. That means that for the first frame $m = 0$ the initial condition is a user-defined signed distance function φ_0 and for the subsequent $M - 1$ frames the initial condition is automatically given by the steady state solution of the previous frame $\varphi_{ss}^{(m-1)}$. We found that the best results are obtained by considering a starting frame to be the one corresponding to the early diastole, where the mitral valve is completely opened, and to continue the segmentation for half the cardiac cycle in the positive time direction and for the remaining half in the negative time direction, namely:

$$\varphi_0^{(M/2)} = \varphi_0$$
$$\varphi_0^{(m)} = \varphi_{ss}^{(m-1)}, m = (M/2 + 1) \ldots M$$
$$\varphi_0^{(m-1)} = \varphi_{ss}^{(m)}, m = (M/2 - 1) \ldots 0$$

The result of applying this procedure on a time sequence of $2D$ echocardiographic images is shown in Figures 3.9-3.10. In Figures 3.11-3.12, we follow the same procedure and show results from echocardiographic data acquired with the real-time volumetric ultrasound imaging system (RT3DE) developed by Volumetrics Medical Inc.. This system allows 3D acquisition of dynamic structures in real-time. It involves a 2D array transducer that generates a pyramidal burst of ultrasound whose returning signals are utilized to create the 3D image. Volumetrics operates with 2.5-3.5 MHz transducers. The transducer is a matrix array of 43x43 square piezoelectric crystal elements each measuring 0.3x0.3 mm. The system has 64 transmission channels and 64 receiving channels, and therefore only a small part of the transducer elements is used in two independent and different transmission and reception apertures. It is based on a parallel reception processing mode scheme to improve the data acquisition rate for volumetric imaging. These clinical images were obtained from transthoracic windows using an apical 4-chamber view as an original guiding reference and a 2-chamber view for orthogonal images.

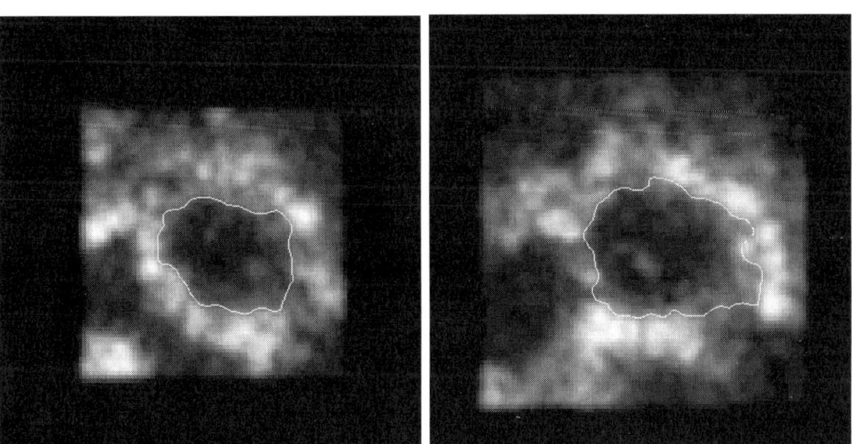

Fig. 3.9. Segmentation of the ventricular chamber from a sequence of time varying echocardiograms. Frames #14 and #15.

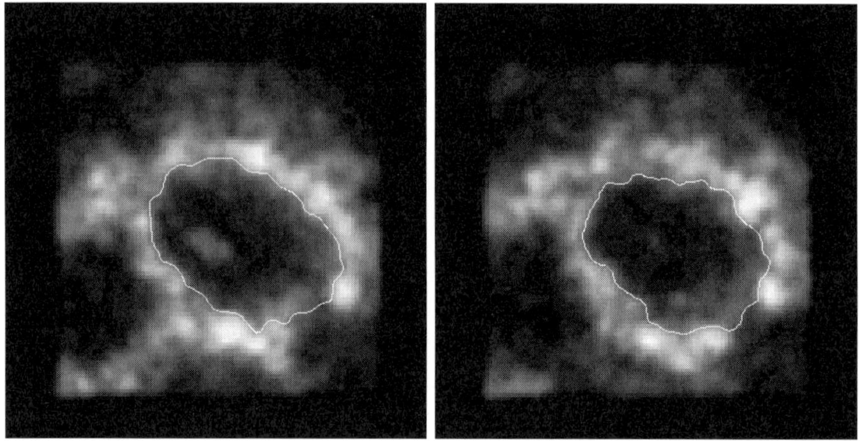

Fig. 3.10. Segmentation of the ventricular chamber from a sequence of time varying echocardiograms. Frames #19 and #20.

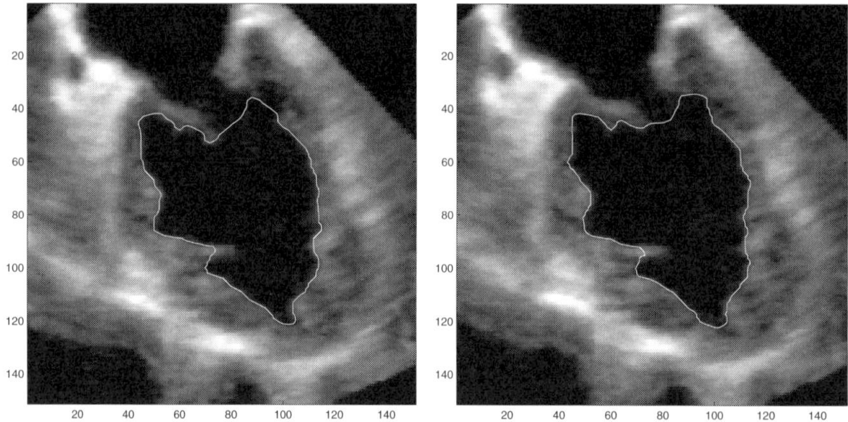

Fig. 3.11. Segmentation of the ventricular chamber from a sequence time varying $2D$ echocardiographic images. Frames #7 and #8.

3.7 $3D$ Echocardiography

We want to accurately extract the $3D$ ventricular shape by retaining the advantages such as easy initialization in $2D$ segmentation and also the regularization properties of a real $3D$ shape extraction method [16,17]. We again face the same difficulty that the edge map in $3D$ is both noisy and has many gaps. In addition, in $3D$ it is also problematic for the user to specify an initial model that is reasonably close to the final surface. With this in mind we propose a chain of models to achieve our goal.

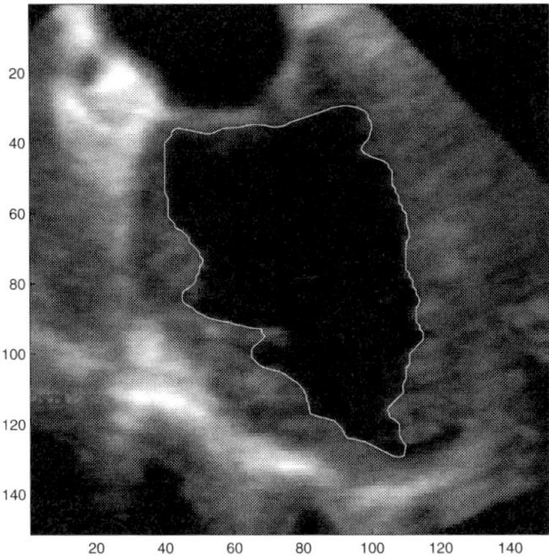

Fig. 3.12. Segmentation of the ventricular chamber from a sequence time varying $2D$ echocardiographic images. Frame #11

First, consider a $3D$ echocardiographic image I_V as a stack of 2-dimensional slices $I_V^{(l)}, l = 0 \ldots L$. As in the $2D + time$ case we apply a sequence of $2D$ segmentation steps using the following model:

$$\varphi_t^{(l)} = g^{(l)} K^{(l)} |\nabla \varphi^{(l)}| + \beta \nabla g^{(l)} \cdot \nabla \varphi^{(l)} \tag{3.21}$$

$$g^{(l)}(x) = \frac{1}{1 + (|\nabla I_{V_{GS}}^{(l)}(x)|/\alpha)^2} \tag{3.22}$$

with the initial conditions:

$$\varphi_0^{(l_0)} = \varphi_0$$
$$\varphi_0^{(l)} = \varphi_{ss}^{(l-1)}, l = l_0 \ldots L$$
$$\varphi_0^{(l-1)} = \varphi_{ss}^{(l)}, l = l_0 \ldots 0$$

where l_0 is a suitable slice. The best results are obtained when l_0 is a long axis view that contains both the mitral valve and the apex. At the end of this stage we have a set of $2D$ contours when stacked on top of each other will provide a good initial guess to start the $3D$ shape extraction problem.

Therefore, we now consider the entire $3D$ image and perform a real $3D$ segmentation by evolving the embedding $\phi : \Omega \times [0, T] \rightarrow R, \Omega \subset R^3$, with the flow:

$$\phi_t = gH|\nabla \phi| + \beta \nabla g \cdot \nabla \phi$$

$$g(x) = \frac{1}{1 + (|\nabla I_{V_{GS}}(x)|/\alpha)^2} \tag{3.23}$$

with the initial condition given by the union of the previous set of $2D$ segmentation results, i.e. $\phi(0) = U\varphi_{ss}^{(l)}, l = 0 \ldots L$.

The mean curvature H can be expressed as a function of the embedding as follows:

$$H = \nabla \cdot \frac{\nabla \phi}{|\nabla \phi|} = \frac{\left\{ \begin{array}{c} (\phi_{yy} + \phi_{zz})\phi_x^2 + (\phi_{xx} + \phi_{zz})\phi_y^2 + (\phi_{xx} + \phi_{yy})\phi_z^2 \\ -2\phi_x\phi_y\phi_{xy} - 2\phi_x\phi_z\phi_{xz} - 2\phi_y\phi_z\phi_{yz} \end{array} \right\}}{(\phi_x^2 + \phi_y^2 + \phi_z^2)^{(3/2)}} \quad (3.24)$$

To discretize Eqn. 3.23 consider a uniform grid in space-time (t, x, y, z); then the grid will be the points $(t_n, x_i, y_j, z_k) = (n\Delta t, i\Delta x, j\Delta y, k\Delta z)$. Then the first order scheme that approximates Eqn. 3.23 is

$$\phi_{ijk}^{n+1} = \phi_{ijk}^n + \Delta t \left[\begin{array}{c} [g_{ijk}H_{ijk}^n(D_{ijk}^{0x^2} + D_{ijk}^{0y^2} + D_{ijk}^{0z^2})^{1/2}] \\ - \left\{ \begin{array}{l} [max(g_{ijk}^{0x},0)D_{ijk}^{-x} + min(g_{ijk}^{0x},0)D_{ijk}^{+x} \\ +max(g_{ijk}^{0y},0)D_{ijk}^{-y} + min(g_{ijk}^{0y},0)D_{ijk}^{+y} \\ +max(g_{ijk}^{0z},0)D_{ijk}^{-z} + min(g_{ijk}^{0z},0)D_{ijk}^{+z}] \end{array} \right\} \end{array} \right] \quad (3.25)$$

using the same notation as before. A demonstration of this scheme is shown in Figure 3.13. The picture on the left is a rendering of the initial surface constructed by assembling all the individual $2D$ contours. This shape is then regularized and drawn towards the $3D$ edge map by solving Eqn. 3.23 for a few time steps; the result is depicted in the right picture.

Next, we compare the volume measurement we obtain from our $3D$ segmentation to that of experimentally computed values on a couple of sheep heart data sets. The echocardiographic data was obtained from sheep hearts; for details on data acquisition and experimental heart volume computation, the reader is referred to the work of Pin $et.$ al [21,22]. The volume figures on two sheep hearts according to [21,22] are 39.0 and 35.7 cm^3, and the volume figures we obtain by first extracting the $3D$ surfaces from corresponding echocardiograms is 42.2 and 35.4 cm^3, i.e. an error of 7.6 % and 0.8 % respectively. Some cross-sections of those surfaces is shown in Figure 3.14.

3.8 $3D + time$ Echocardiography

Finally, let us consider a $3D$ sequence of echocardiographic images $I_{VT}^{(m)}, m = 0 \ldots M$. To segment the ventricular shape from the entire sequence, we adopt the same strategy as we did for time varying $2D$ seqence and apply the following flow:

$$\phi_t^{(m)} = g^{(m)} H^{(m)} |\nabla \phi^{(m)}| + \beta \nabla g^{(m)} \cdot \nabla \phi^{(m)} \quad (3.26)$$

$$g^{(m)}(x) = \frac{1}{1 + (|\nabla I_{VT_{GS}}^{(m)}(x)|/\alpha)^2} \quad (3.27)$$

This equation is solved with appropriate initial conditions for each time frame. We applied this scheme to a time varying sequence of echocardiograms

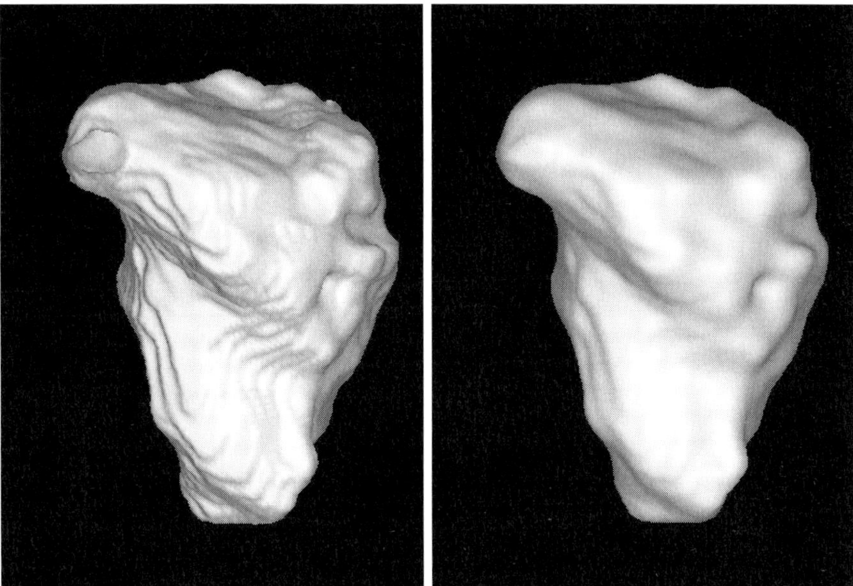

Fig. 3.13. Extraction of the ventricular chamber in $3D$ echocardiography. Left: segmentation of the $3D$ image as a spatial sequence of $2D$ images. Right: full $3D$ shape segmentation by using the volume on the left as initial condition for the 3D level set Eq. 3.23.

and computed the volume of the left ventricular shape while the heart is in a cardiac cycle. The plot of the computed volume is shown in Figure 3.15. It is now possible to reliably compute quantities like the ejection fraction from noisy echocardiograms.

3.9   Conclusions

We presented a geometry-based partial differential equation (PDE) approach for filtering and segmentation of echocardiographic images. The method allows edge-preserving image smoothing and a semi-automatic segmentation of the heart chambers. This approach uses regularization to fill in the edge-gaps and improves edge fidelity. A numerical scheme for solving the proposed PDE is carried out from level set methods. Results on human in vivo acquired $2D$, $2D + time$, $3D$, and $3D + time$ echocardiographic images have been shown.

Acknowledgements

The authors would like to thank B. Mumm at Tomtec for supplying the sequence of 3D Echo data, the Cleveland Clinic Foundation for the RT3DE data and R. Pini for providing the sheep heart data for the validation. Thanks to M. Borsari and C. Corsi for their help in manual segmentation and software

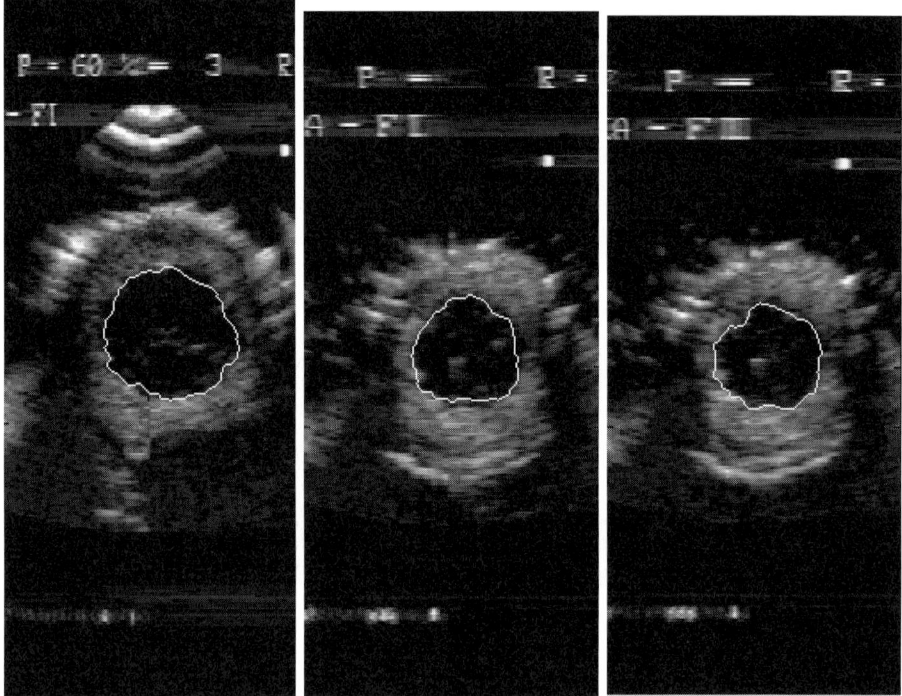

Fig. 3.14. Heart shape extraction and volume comparison from $3D$ images of sheep hearts.

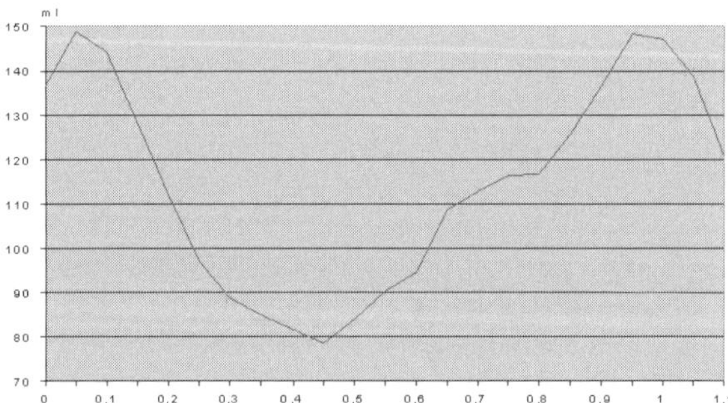

Fig. 3.15. The estimated ventricular volume during an entire cardiac cycle

development. The work was supported by the Office of Energy Research, Office of Computational and Technology Research, Mathematical, Information and Computational Science Division, Applied Mathematical Sciences Subprogram, of the U.S. Department of Energy, under Contract No. DE-AC03-76SF00098.

References

1. D. Adalsteinsson and J. A. Sethian: A fast level set method for propagating interfaces, in *J. Comp. Phys.*, Vol. 118(2), pp. 269–277, May 1995.
2. L. Alvarez, F. Guichard, P. L. Lions, and J. M. Morel: Axioms and fundamental equations of image processing, *Arch. Rational Mechanics* **123**, 1993.
3. W. Bommer, L. Weinert, A. Neumann, J. Neef, D. Mason, A. Demaria: *Determination of right atrial and right ventricular size by two-dimensional echocardiography*, Circulation, pp. 60-91 (1979)
4. V. Caselles, F. Catte. T. Coll, F. Dibos: A geometric model for active contours, *Numerische Mathematik*, Vol. 66, pp. 1–31, 1993.
5. V. Caselles, R. Kimmel, and G. Sapiro: Geodesic active contours, in *Proc. ICCV'95*, Cambridge, MA 1995.
6. L.D Cohen: *On active contour models and balloons* CVGIP:Image Understanding vol. 53, pag. 211-218.
7. I. Cohen, L.D Cohen, N. Ayache: *Using deformable surfaces to segment 3D images and infer differential structure* CVGIP:Image Understanding vol. 56, pag. 242-263.
8. M. Grayson: The heat equation shrinks embedded plane curves to round points, *J. Differential Geometry* **26**, 1987, pp. 285-314.
9. A.Handlovičová, K.Mikula, A.Sarti: *Numerical solution of parabolic equations related to level set formulation of mean curvature flow*, Computing and Visualization in Science (1998)
10. C. Lamberti, F. Sgallari: *Edge detection and velocity field for the analysis of heart motion*, Digital Signal Processing 91, Elsevier (Editors V. Cappellini, A.G. Costantinides) pp. 603-608 (1991)
11. W.E. Lorensen, H.E. Cline: *Marching cubes: a high resolution 3D surface construction algorithm*, Computer Graph., vol. 21, pp. 163-169 (1987)
12. M. Kass, A. Witkin, D. Terzopoulos: *Snakes: Active contour models*, International Journal of Computer Vision, vol. 1, pp. 321-331, 1988
13. R. Malladi, J.A. Sethian, B.C. Vemuri: A topology-independent shape modeling scheme, in *SPIE: Geometric Methods in Computer Vision II*, Vol. 2031, pp. 246–258, 1993.
14. R. Malladi, J. A. Sethian and B. C. Vemuri: Shape modeling with front propagation: A level set approach, *IEEE Trans. on PAMI* **17**, 1995, pp. 158-175.
15. R. Malladi and J. A. Sethian: Image processing: Flows under Min/Max curvature and mean curvature, in *Graphical Models and Image Processing*, Vol. 58(2), pp. 127–141, March 1996.
16. R. Malladi and J. A. Sethian: Level set methods for curvature flow, image enchancement, and shape recovery in medical images, in *Visualization and Mathematics: Experiments, Simulations, and Environments*, Eds. H. C. Hege, K. Polthier, pp. 329–345, Springer Verlag, Heidelberg, 1997.
17. R. Malladi and J. A. Sethian: A real-time algorithm for medical shape recovery, in *Proceedings of ICCV '98*, pp. 304–310, Mumbai India, January 1998.
18. K.Mikula, A.Sarti, C.Lamberti: Geometrical diffusion in 3D echocardiography, *Proc. of ALGORITMY '97- Conference on Scientific Computing*, West Tatra Mountains, Slovakia, 1997.
19. N. K. Nordstrom: Variational edge detection, *PhD dissertation* , Department of electrical engineering, University of California, Berkeley, 1990

20. S. J. Osher and J. A. Sethian: Fronts propagation with curvature dependent speed: Algorithms based on Hamilton-Jacobi formulations, *Journal of Computational Physics* **79**, 1988, pp. 12-49.

21. Pini R, Giannazzo G, Di Bari M, Innocenti F, Rega L, Casolo G, and Devereux RB: Transthoracic three-dimensional echocardiographic reconstruction of left and right ventricles: In vitro validation and comparison with magnetic resonance imaging,*American Heart Journal*, 133: pp. 221–229, 1997.

22. Pini R, Giannazzo G, Di Bari M, Innocenti F, Marchionni N, Gori A, and Devereux RB: Left ventricular volume determination by 3-D echocardiographic volume imaging and biplane angiography, *Journal of Noninvasive Cardiology*, 3, pp. 46–51, 1999.

23. Bart M. ter Haar Romeny(Ed.): *Geometry-driven diffusion in computer vision*, Kluwer Academic Press, 1994.

24. G. Sapiro: Color snakes, Hewlett-Packard Lab. tech report, 1995.

25. G. Sapiro, R. Kimmel, D. Shaked, B. B. Kimia, and A. M. Bruckstein: Implementing continuous-scale morphology via curve evolution, *Pattern Recognition*, Vol. 26(9), pp. 1363–1372, 1993.

26. Sarti, A., Mikula, K., Sgallari, F.: Nonlinear multiscale analysis of 3D echocardiographic sequences. IEEE Transactions on Medical Imaging **18**, No. 6 (1999) 453–466

27. Sarti,A., Ortiz de Solorzano,C., Lockett, S. and Malladi, R.: A Geometric Model for 3-D Confocal Image Analysis. IEEE Transactions on Biomedical Engineering **45**, No. 12, (2000), 1600–1610

28. Sarti,A., Malladi,R., Sethian,J.A.: Subjective Surfaces: A Method for Completing Missing Boundaries. Proceedings of the National Academy of Sciences of the United States of America,Vol 12, N.97, pag. 6258-6263, 2000.

29. Sarti,A., Malladi,R., Sethian,J.A.: Subjective Surfaces: A Geometric Model for Boundary Completion, submitted to International Journal of Computer Vision, 2000.

30. Sarti,A., Malladi,R.: A geometric level set model for ultrasounds analysis, LBNL-44442, University of California, Berkeley, 1999.

31. Sarti,A., Wiegmann,A.: Edges are image discontinuities–fast edge enhancement based on explicit-jump multiscale analysis, LBNL-42373, University of California, Berkeley, 1999.

32. J. A. Sethian: A review of recent numerical algorithms for hypersurfaces moving with curvature dependent flows, *J. Differential Geometry* **31**, 1989, pp. 131-161.

33. J. A. Sethian: *Level set methods: Evolving interfaces in geometry, fluid mechanics, computer vision, and material science*, Cambridge University Press, 1997.

34. W. Shroeder, K. Martin, B. Lorensen: *The visualization Toolkit*, Prentice Hall PTR., New Jersey (1996)

35. S.Shutilov: *Fundamental Physics of Ultrasounds*, Gordon and Breach , New York, 1988

36. N. Sochen, R. Kimmel, and R. Malladi: A General Framework for Low Level Vision, in *IEEE Transactions on Image Processing*, special issue on PDEs and Geometry-Driven Diffusion in Image Processing and Analysis, Vol. 7, No. 3, pp. 310–318, March 1998.

4 Active Contour and Segmentation Models using Geometric PDE's for Medical Imaging *

T. F. Chan and L. A. Vese

Department of Mathematics, University of California, Los Angeles,
405 Hilgard Avenue, Los Angeles, CA 90095-1555, U.S.A.
E-mail: chan@ipam.ucla.edu, lvese@math.ucla.edu

Abstract. This paper is devoted to the analysis and the extraction of information from bio-medical images. The proposed technique is based on object and contour detection, curve evolution and segmentation. We present a particular active contour model for 2D and 3D images, formulated using the level set method, and based on a 2-phase piecewise-constant segmentation. We then show how this model can be generalized to segmentation of images with more than two segments. The techniques used are based on the Mumford-Shah [21] model. By the proposed models, we can extract in addition measurements of the detected objects, such as average intensity, perimeter, area, or volume. Such informations are useful when in particular a time evolution of the subject is known, or when we need to make comparisons between different subjects, for instance between a normal subject and an abnormal one. Finally, all these will give more informations about the dynamic of a disease, or about how the human body growths. We illustrate the efficiency of the proposed models by calculations on two-dimensional and three-dimensional bio-medical images.

4.1 Introduction

Techniques of image processing and data analysis are more and more used in the medical field. Mathematical algorithms of feature extraction, modelization and measurements can exploit the data to detect pathology in an individual or patient group, the evolution of the disease, or to compare a normal subject to an abnormal one.

In this paper, we show how the active contour model without edges introduced in [7], and its extension to segmentation of images from [8], can be applied to medical images. The benefits of these algorithms can be summarized in: automatically detecting interior contours, robust with respect to noise, ability to detect and represent complex topologies (boundaries, segments), and finally, extraction of geometric measurements, such as length, area, volume, intensity, of a detected contour, surface or region, respectively. These informations can be later used to study the evolution in time of a disease (a growing tumor), or to compare two different subjects, usually a normal one and an abnormal one.

* This work was supported in part by ONR Contract N00014-96-1-0277 and NSF Contract DMS-9973341.

In active contours, the basic idea is to evolve a curve C in a given image u_0, and to stop the evolution when the curve meets an object or a boundary of the image. In order to stop the curve on the desired objects, classical models use the magnitude of the gradient of the image, to detect the boundaries of the object. Therefore, these models can detect only edges defined by gradient. Some of these classical models suffer from other limitations: the initial curve has to surround the objects to be detected, and interior contours cannot be detected automatically. We refer the reader to [9], [3], [16], [17] [18], [4], [10], for a few examples of active contour models based on the gradient for the stopping criteria.

The active contour model that we will use here [7], is different than the classical ones, because it is not based on the gradient (a local information) for the stopping criteria. Instead, it is based on a global segmentation of the image, and it has the advantages mentioned above. For the implementation of the active contour model , the level set method of S. Osher and J. Sethian [22] has been efficiently used. We have also extended this model to segment images, based on the piecewise-constant Mumford-Shah model [21], using a particular multiphase level set formulation [8]. This formulation allows for multiple segments, triple junctions, complex topologies and in addition, compared with other multiphase level set formulations, the problems of vacuum and overlap of phases cannot arise.

Before going further, we would like to refer the reader to other works on segmentation using Mumford-Shah techniques: [1], [2], [5], [6], [12], [19], [20], [23], [25], [26], [28], [30], [31], and to related works with applications to medical imagery: [27], [14], [15], [11], [24], [13].

We will first recall the active contour model without edges from [7], and its extension to segmentation of images [8]. Then, we will illustrate how these geometric PDE models can be applied to segmentation of medical images.

4.2   Description of the Models

Let us first introduce our notations. Let $\Omega \subset I\!R^n \to I\!R$ be an open and bounded set, and let $u_0 : \overline{\Omega} \to I\!R$ be a given image. In our case, we will consider $n = 2$ (plane images), and $n = 3$ (volumetric images), and $x \in I\!R^n$ denotes an arbitrary point. Let $C \subset \Omega$ be a hyper-surface, as the boundary of an open subset ω of Ω, i.e. ω is open, $\omega \subset \Omega$ and $C = \partial\omega$. We call "$inside(C)$" the region given by ω, and "$outside(C)$" the region given by $\Omega \setminus \overline{\omega}$. We recall that $\mathcal{H}^{n-1}$ denotes the $(n-1)$-dimensional Hausdorff measure in $I\!R^n$. For $n = 2$, $\mathcal{H}^{n-1}(C)$ gives the length of the curve C, and for $n = 3$, $\mathcal{H}^{n-1}(C)$ gives the area of the surface C.

In this paper, we consider the problem of active contours and object detection, via the level set method [22] and Mumford-Shah segmentation [21]. Giving an initial hyper-surface C, we evolve it under some constraints, in order to detect objects in the image u_0. In addition, we also obtain a segmentation of the image, given by the connected components of $\Omega \setminus C$ and the averages of u_0 in these regions. Finally, we would like to extract more informations, in the form of geometrical measurements for the detected objects.

We introduce an energy based segmentation, as a particular case of the minimal partition problem of Mumford-Shah [21]. As in [7], we denote by c_1 and c_2 two unknown constants, representing the averages of the image u_0 inside C and outside C, respectively. A variant of the model introduced in [7], but generalized to n dimensions, is:

$$\inf_{c_1, c_2, C} F(c_1, c_2, C), \tag{4.1}$$

where, using the above notations,

$$F(c_1, c_2, C) = \lambda_1 \int_{inside(C)} (u_0(x) - c_1)^2 dx + \lambda_2 \int_{outside(C)} (u_0(x) - c_2)^2 dx$$
$$+ \mu \mathcal{H}^{n-1}(C) + \nu \mathcal{L}^n(inside(C)).$$

Here, $\mathcal{L}^n$ denotes the Lebesgue measure in $\mathbb{R}^n$. For $n = 2$, $\mathcal{L}^2(\omega)$ denotes the area of ω, and for $n = 3$, $\mathcal{L}^3(\omega)$ denotes the volume of ω. The coefficients $\lambda_1, \lambda_2, \mu$ and ν are fixed non-negative constants.

Minimizing the above energy with respect to c_1, c_2 and C, leads to an active contour model, based on segmentation. It looks for the best simplest approximation of the image taking only two values, c_1 and c_2, and the active contour is the boundary between the two corresponding regions. One of the regions represents the objects to be detected, and the other region gives the background. We note that, when $\lambda_1 = \lambda_2 = 1$ and $\nu = 0$, the minimization of the above energy is a particular case of the piecewise-constant Mumford-Shah model for segmentation [21].

For the evolving curve C, we use an implicit representation given by the level set method of S. Osher and J. Sethian [22], because it has many advantages, comparing with an explicit parameterization: it allows for automatic change of topology, cusps, merging and breaking, and the calculations are made on a fix rectangular grid. In this framework, as in [22], a hyper-surface $C \in \Omega$ is represented implicitly via a Lipschitz function $\phi : \Omega \to \mathbb{R}$, such that: $C = \{x \in \Omega | \phi(x) = 0\}$. Also, ϕ needs to have opposite signs on each side of C. For instance, we can choose $\phi(x) > 0$ inside C (i.e. in ω), and $\phi(x) < 0$ outside C (i.e. in $\Omega \setminus \bar{\omega}$).

As in [7], also following [29], we can formulate the above active contour model in terms of level sets. We therefore replace the unknown variable C by the unknown variable ϕ. Using the Heaviside function H defined by:

$$H(z) = \begin{cases} 1, & \text{if } z \geq 0 \\ 0, & \text{if } z < 0, \end{cases}$$

we express the terms in the energy F in the following way:

$$F(c_1, c_2, \phi) = \lambda_1 \int_{\phi>0} (u_0(x) - c_1)^2 dx + \lambda_2 \int_{\phi<0} (u_0(x) - c_2)^2 dx$$
$$+ \mu \mathcal{H}^{n-1}(C) + \nu \mathcal{L}^n(C),$$

or

$$F(c_1, c_2, \phi) = \lambda_1 \int_\Omega (u_0(x) - c_1)^2 H(\phi(x)) dx$$
$$+\lambda_2 \int_\Omega (u_0(x) - c_2)^2 (1 - H(\phi(x)) dx + \mu \int_\Omega |\nabla H(\phi(x))| + \nu \int_\Omega H(\phi(x)) dx.$$

Considering H_ε and δ_ε any C^1 approximations and regularizations of the Heaviside function H and Delta function δ_0, as $\varepsilon \to 0$, and with $H'_\varepsilon = \delta_\varepsilon$, and minimizing the energy with respect to c_1, c_2, and ϕ, we obtain:

$$c_1 = \frac{\int_\Omega u_0(x) H(\phi(x)) dx}{\int_\Omega H(\phi(x)) dx}, \quad c_2 = \frac{\int_\Omega u_0(x)(1 - H(\phi(x))) dx}{\int_\Omega (1 - H(\phi(x))) dx},$$

and

$$\frac{\partial \phi}{\partial t} = \delta_\varepsilon(\phi) \left[\mathrm{div}\left(\frac{\nabla \phi}{|\nabla \phi|} \right) - \lambda_1 (u_0 - c_1)^2 + \lambda_2 (u_0 - c_2)^2 - \nu \right].$$

We see that c_1 and c_2 are the averages of the image u_0 inside C and outside C respectively. Solving the equation in ϕ by an iterative scheme, we implicitly move the curve C toward boundaries in the image. The motion of the curve is governed by the mean curvature $\mathrm{div}\left(\frac{\nabla \phi}{|\nabla \phi|} \right)$ and by terms depending on u_0. In the end, we also obtain a two-phase segmentation of the image, given by $u(x) = c_1 H(\phi(x)) + c_2 (1 - H(\phi(x)))$.

This model can be extended to the general piecewise-constant Mumford-Shah segmentation model [21] (when we look for more than two segments), originally proposed in two dimensions. It minimizes the energy

$$F^{MS}(u, C) = \sum_i \int_{\Omega_i} (u_0(x) - c_i)^2 dx + \mu \mathcal{H}^{n-1}(C), \qquad (4.2)$$

where $u = c_i$ inside each connected component of $\Omega \setminus C$.

In order to find a piecewise-constant approximation of u_0 based on the above Mumford-Shah model and level sets, we propose a multiphase level set representation, which allows for multiple segments and triple junctions. The basic idea is to use several level set functions. In [29] for instance, one level set function is associated to each phase. But in our formulation, we considerably reduce the number of level set functions, in the following way. As we have seen, using one level set function ϕ, we can partition the domain Ω in up to two disjoint regions, given by $\{\phi > 0\}$ and $\{\phi < 0\}$. Using two level set functions ϕ_1, ϕ_2, we can partition the domain in up to four disjoint regions, given by $\{\phi_1 > 0, \phi_2 > 0\}$, $\{\phi_1 > 0, \phi_2 < 0\}$, $\{\phi_1 < 0, \phi_2 > 0\}$, and $\{\phi_1 < 0, \phi_2 < 0\}$; and so on, using n level set functions $\phi_1, ..., \phi_n$, we can define up to 2^n regions or phases. These are disjoint (no overlap) and form a covering of Ω (no vacuum).

Let us write the associated energy for $n = 2$ level set functions, for instance, for the purpose of illustration (see [8] for more general cases):

$$F(c, \Phi) = \int_\Omega (u_0(x) - c_{11})^2 H(\phi_1(x)) H(\phi_2(x)) dx$$

$$+ \int_\Omega (u_0(x) - c_{10})^2 H(\phi_1(x))(1 - H(\phi_2(x))) dx$$

$$+ \int_\Omega (u_0(x) - c_{01})^2 (1 - H(\phi_1(x))) H(\phi_2(x)) dx$$

$$+ \int_\Omega (u_0(x) - c_{00})^2 (1 - H(\phi_1(x)))(1 - H(\phi_2(x))) dx$$

$$+ \mu \int_\Omega |\nabla H(\phi_1(x))| + \mu \int_\Omega |\nabla H(\phi_2(x))|,$$

where $c = (c_{11}, c_{10}, c_{01}, c_{00})$, $\Phi = (\phi_1, \phi_2)$.

With these notations, we can express the image-function u as:

$$u(x) = c_{11} H(\phi_1(x)) H(\phi_2(x)) + c_{10} H(\phi_1(x))(1 - H(\phi_2(x)))$$
$$+ c_{01}(1 - H(\phi_1(x))) H(\phi_2(x)) + c_{00}(1 - H(\phi_1(x)))(1 - H(\phi_2(x))).$$

The Euler-Lagrange equations obtained by minimizing $F(c, \Phi)$ with respect to c and Φ are:

$$\begin{cases} c_{11} = mean(u_0) \text{ in } \{\phi_1 > 0, \phi_2 > 0\} \\ c_{10} = mean(u_0) \text{ in } \{\phi_1 > 0, \phi_2 < 0\} \\ c_{01} = mean(u_0) \text{ in } \{\phi_1 < 0, \phi_2 > 0\} \\ c_{00} = mean(u_0) \text{ in } \{\phi_1 < 0, \phi_2 < 0\}, \end{cases} \tag{4.3}$$

$$\frac{\partial \phi_1}{\partial t} = \delta_\varepsilon(\phi_1)\left\{\mu \mathrm{div}\left(\frac{\nabla \phi_1}{|\nabla \phi_1|}\right) - \left[\left((u_0 - c_{11})^2 - (u_0 - c_{01})^2\right) H(\phi_2) \right. \tag{4.4}$$

$$\left. + \left((u_0 - c_{10})^2 - (u_0 - c_{00})^2\right)(1 - H(\phi_2))\right]\right\}, \tag{4.5}$$

and

$$\frac{\partial \phi_2}{\partial t} = \delta_\varepsilon(\phi_2)\left\{\mu \mathrm{div}\left(\frac{\nabla \phi_2}{|\nabla \phi_2|}\right) - \left[\left((u_0 - c_{11})^2 - (u_0 - c_{01})^2\right) H(\phi_1) \right. \tag{4.6}$$

$$\left. + \left((u_0 - c_{10})^2 - (u_0 - c_{00})^2\right)(1 - H(\phi_1))\right]\right\}. \tag{4.7}$$

We note that the equations in $\Phi = (\phi_1, \phi_2)$ are governed by both mean curvature and jump of the data energy terms across the boundary.

After each calculation, we can extract the length or the area of the evolving contour or surface using the formula $\int_\Omega |\nabla H(\phi(x))|dx$, the area or the volume of the detected objects (integrating the characteristic functions of each component of the partition), and the average intensity of the image u_0 inside the object, given by the computed constants.

4.3   Applications to Bio-Medical Images

In this section, we show how the previous active contour model without edges and its extension to segmentation can be applied to medical images. In our numerical results, $\lambda_1 = \lambda_2 = 1$ and $\nu = 0$. The only varying parameter is μ, the coefficient of the length term, which has a scaling role. We will use the notations A_i (or V_i) for the area (or the volume) of the region given by c_i, by L (or L_i) for the perimeter of the same region, and by A the area of the active surface in 3D, and so on. In most of the experimental results we have $\lambda_1 = \lambda_2 = 1$ and $\nu = 0$, except for those from Figure 2, where $\nu > 0$ and $\lambda_1 > \lambda_2$.

In Figure 1, we consider an image representing bone tissues. We perform the active contour model, and we show the evolving curve, together with the segmented image u, given by c_1 if $\phi > 0$ and c_2 if $\phi < 0$. We illustrate here that interior contours are automatically detected, also that complex shapes can be detected, with blurred boundaries. Here, $\mu = 0.001 \cdot 255^2$, $c_1 = 218$, $c_2 = 115$, $A_1 = 22368$, $A_2 = 17830$, $L = 2171.49$.

In Figure 2, we show how a tumor with blurred boundaries can be detected, in an MRI brain data, using the active contour model without edges.

In Figure 3 we show an active surface ($n = 3$), to detect the boundary in a brain MRI volumetric image. We only show a part of the surface, in a 61x61x61 cube. Again, we can extract the area of the detected surface boundary, and the enclosed volume. In Figure 3 we show cross-sections of the 3D results: the evolving curve in a slice. We also show the final segmentation. Here, $\mu = 0.01 \cdot 255^2$. The final geometric quantities are: $c_1 = 164$, $c_2 = 1$, $V_1 = 304992$, $V_2 = 1194140$, $A = 69682.5$.

Finally, in Figures 5 and 6 we apply the four-phase segmentation model, using two level set functions, again on a MRI brain image. Here, four phases are detected (see Figure 4), and in Figure 5 we show the evolution of the curves, together with the corresponding piecewise-constant segmentations ($\mu = 0.01 \cdot 255^2$, $c_{11} = 45$, $c_{10} = 159$, $c_{01} = 9$, $c_{00} = 103$, $A_{11} = 2572$, $A_{10} = 6656$, $A_{01} = 11401$, $A_{00} = 8874$, $L_{11} = 2063$, $L_{10} = 3017$, $L_{01} = 3749$, $L_{00} = 5250$).

4.4   Concluding Remarks

In this paper, we have shown how the geometric PDE models from [7] and [8] can be applied to segmentation and feature extraction for medical images.

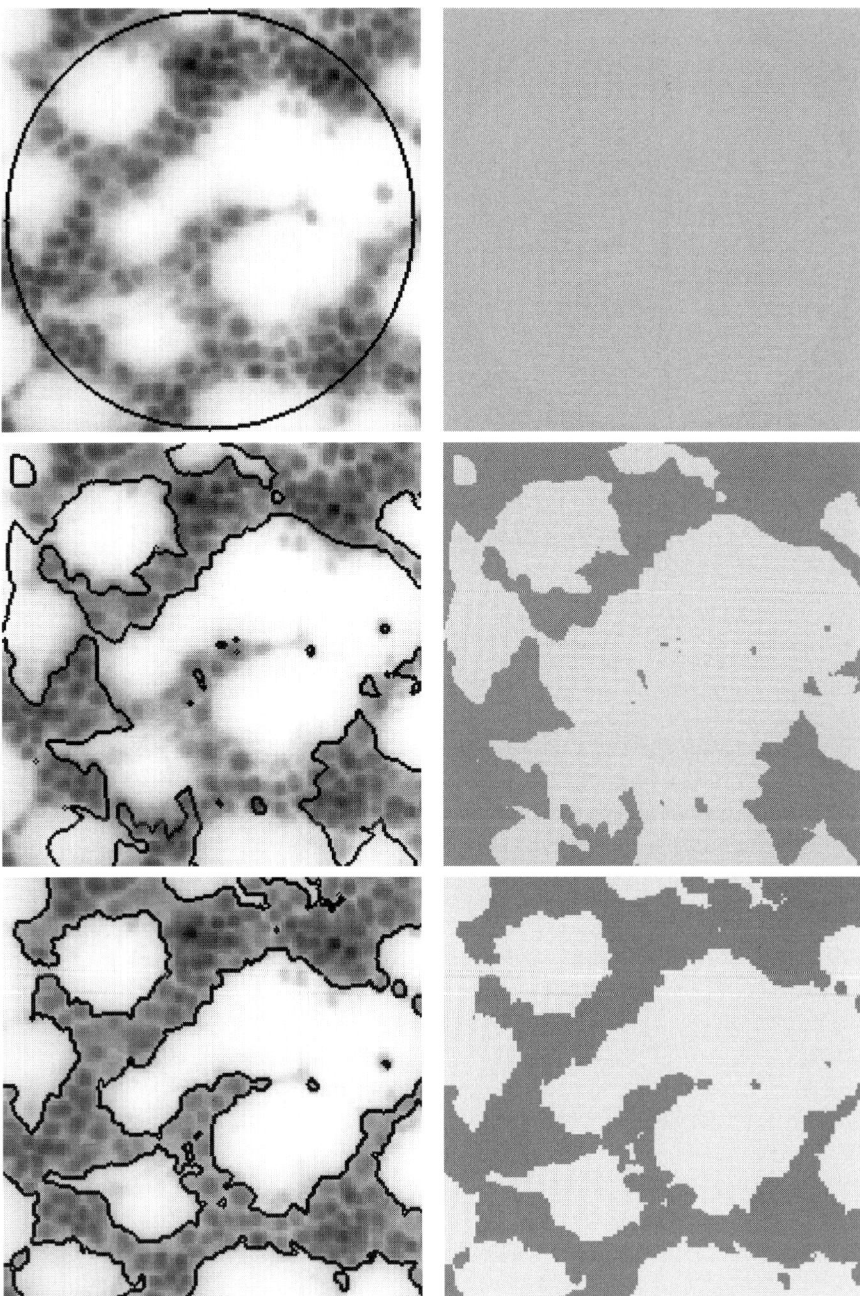

Fig. 4.1. The active contour model applied to a bone tissue image. Left: evolving contour. Right: corresponding two-phase piecewise-constant segmentation. The model can detect blurred edges and interior contours automatically, with automatic change of topology.

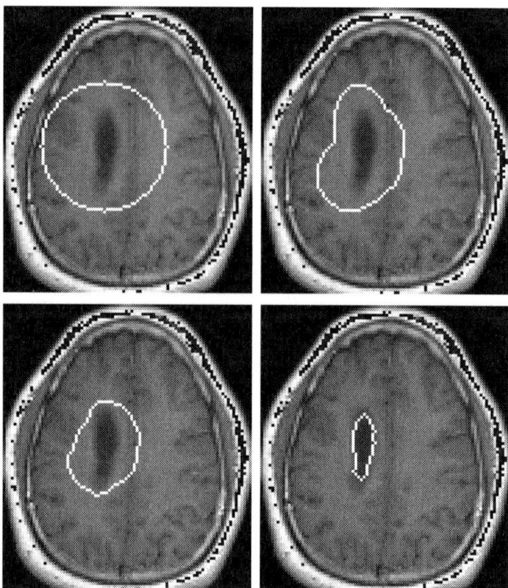

Fig. 4.2. Segmentation of a tumor in an MRI brain data, by the active contour model without edges. We show the evolution of the evolving contour, over the original image.

These methods allow for automatic detection of interior contours, and for segmentation of images with complex topologies into multiple segments, via a new multi-phase level set approach based segmentation. We have illustrated the efficiency of the proposed models by experimental results on 2D and 3D medical images.

Acknowledgments. The authors would like to thank the Editor, Dr. Ravi Malladi, for inviting us to contribute to this book. Also, we would like to thank Dr. Arthur W. Toga and Dr. Paul Thompson, from Laboratory of Neuro Imaging, Department of Neurology, and Dr. Sung-Cheng (Henry) Huang, from Molecular & Medical Pharmacology and Biomathematics, (UCLA School of Medicine), for providing us the MRI brain data, and for very useful discussions.

References

1. Ambrosio, L., Tortorelli, V.M.: Approximation of functionals depending on jumps by elliptic functionals via Γ−convergence. Comm. Pure Appl. Math. **43** (1990) 999–1036.
2. Ambrosio, L., Tortorelli, V.M.: On the Approximation of Free Discontinuity Problems. Bolletino U.M.I. **(7)6-B** (1992) 105–123.
3. Caselles, V., Catté, F., Coll, T., Dibos, F.: A geometric model for active contours in image processing. Numerische Mathematik **66** (1993) 1–31.

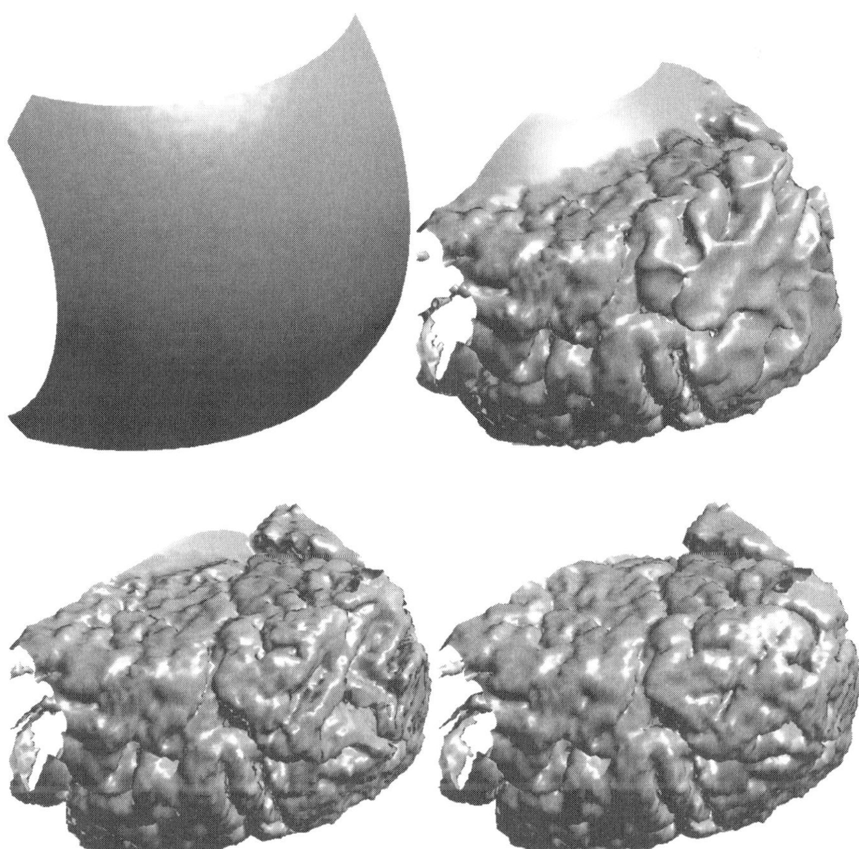

Fig. 4.3. Evolution of an active surface (using the 3D version of the active contour without edges), on a volumetric MRI brain data (we show here only a 61x61x61 cube from the 3D calculations performed on a larger domain, containing the brain.

4. Caselles, V., Kimmel, R., Sapiro, G.: On geodesic active contours. Int. J. of Computer Vision **22/1** (1997) 61–79.
5. Chambolle, A.: Image segmentation by variational methods: Mumford and Shah functional and the discrete approximations. SIAM J. Appl. Math. **55(3)** (1995) 827–863.
6. Chambolle, A.: Finite-differences discretizations of the Mumford-Shah functional. M2AN Math. Model. Numer. Anal. **33(2)** (1999) 261–288.
7. Chan, T., Vese, L.: Active contours without edges. IEEE Transactions on Image Processing. **10/2** (2001) 266–277.
8. Chan, T., Vese, L.: Image segmentation using level sets and the piecewise-constant Mumford-Shah model. UCLA CAM Report 00-14 (2000).
9. Kass, M., Witkin, A., Terzopoulos, D.: Snakes: Active contour models. Int. J. of Computer Vision **1** (1988) 321–331.

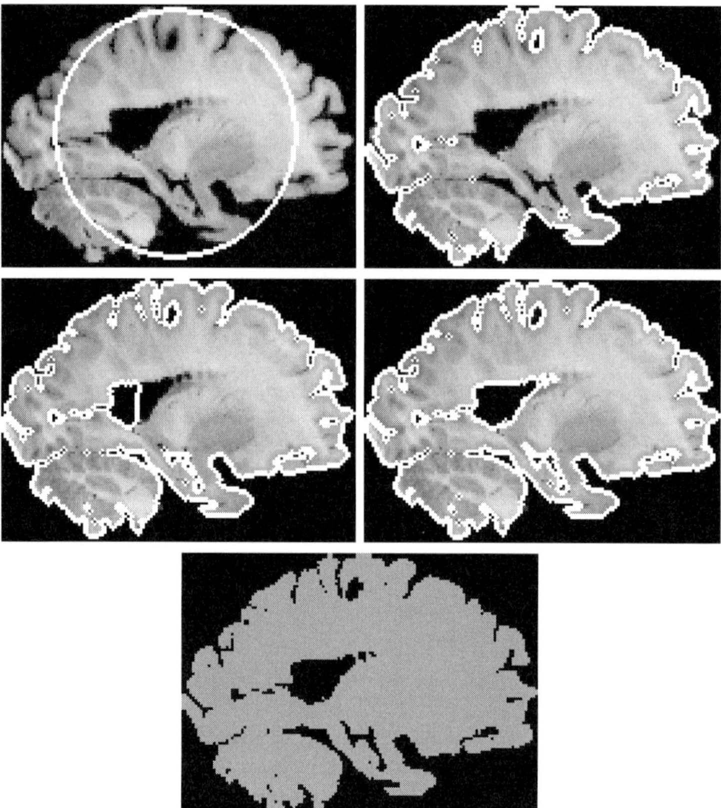

Fig. 4.4. Cross-sections of the previous 3D calculations, showing the evolving contour and the final segmentation on a slice of the volumetric image. We illustrate here how interior boundaries are automatically detected.

10. Kichenassamy, S., Kumar, A., Olver, P., Tannenbaum, A., Yezzi, A.: Gradient flows and geometric active contour models. Proceedings of ICCV, Cambridge, (1995) 810–815.
11. Kimmel, R., Malladi, R., Sochen, N.: Images as Embedded Maps and Minimal Surfaces: Movies, Color, Texture, and Volumetric Medical Images. International Journal of Computer Vision, **39/2** (2000) 111–129.
12. Koepfler, G., Lopez, C., Morel, J.M.: A multiscale algorithm for image segmentation by variational method. SIAM Journal of Numerical Analysis **31-1** (1994) 282–299.
13. Malladi, R., Kimmel, R., Adalsteinsson, D., Caselles, V., Sapiro, G., Sethian, J.A.: A Geometric Approach to Segmentation and Analysis of 3D Medical Images. Proc. of IEEE/SIAM Workshop on Biomedical Image Analysis, San-Francisco, California, (1996).
14. Malladi, R., Sethian, J.A.: A Real-Time Algorithm for Medical Shape Recovery. Proc. of International Conf. on Computer Vision. Mumbai, India (1998) 304–

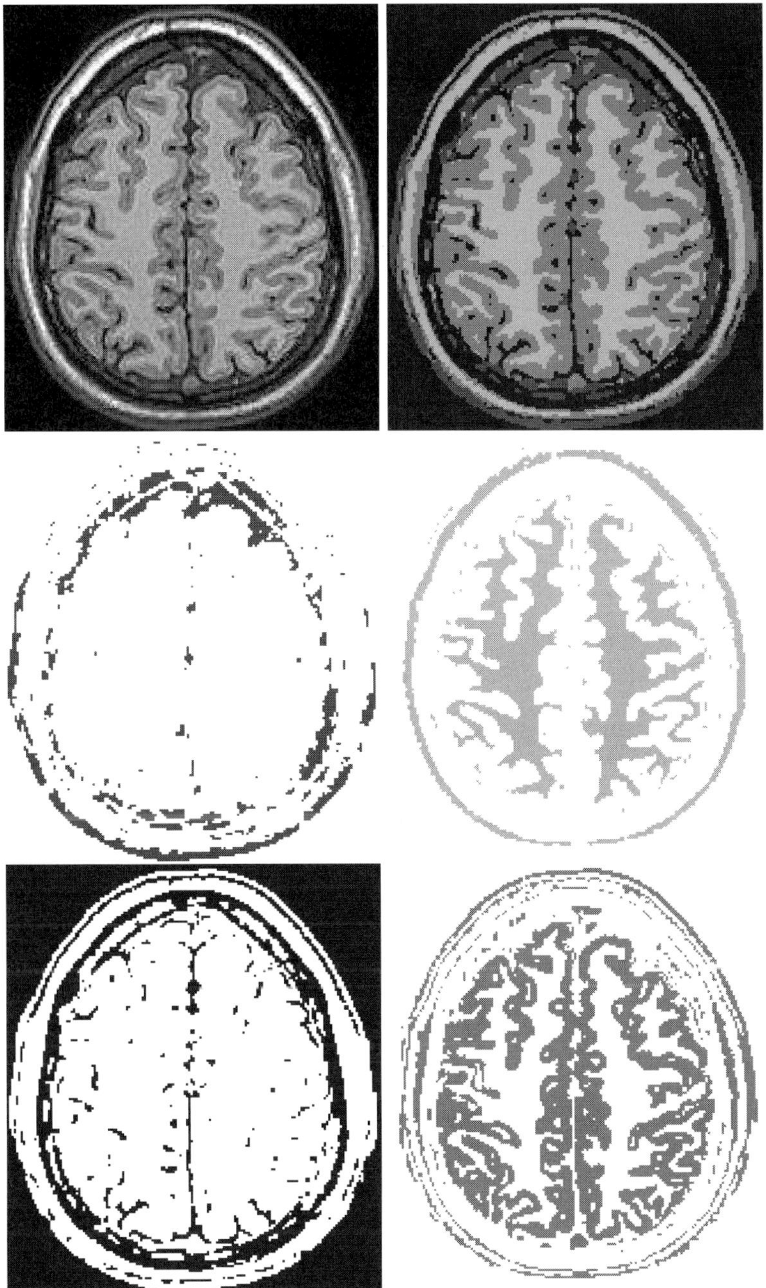

Fig. 4.5. Original & segmented images (top row); final segments (2nd, 3rd rows).

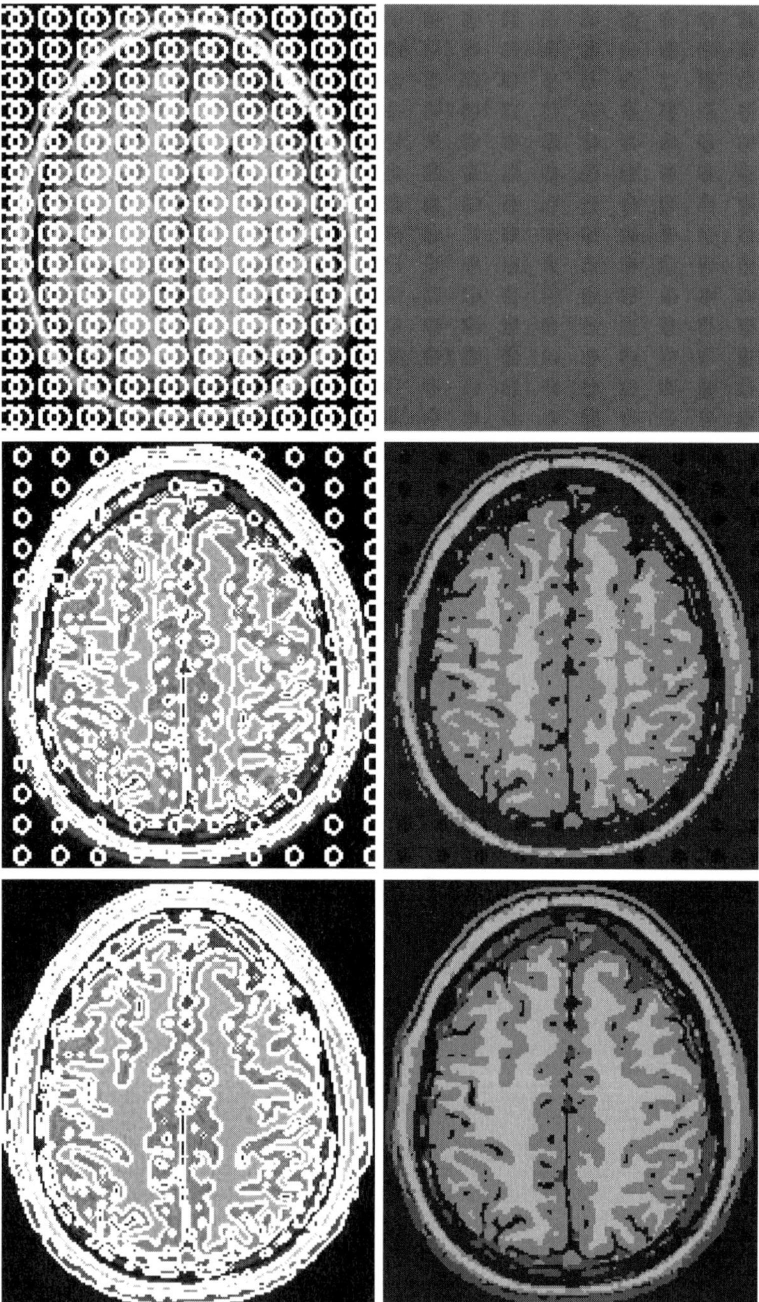

Fig. 4.6. Evolution of the four-phase segmentation model, using two level set functions. Left: the evolving curves. Right: corresponding piecewise-constant segmentations. Initialy, we seed the image with small circles, to obtain a very fast result.

310.

15. Malladi, R., Sethian, J.A.: Level Set Methods for Curvature Flow, Image Enhancement, and Shape Recovery in Medical Images. Visualization and Mathematics, Eds. H. C. Hege, K. Polthier, Springer Verlag, Heidelberg (1997) 329–345.

16. Malladi, R., Sethian, J.A., Vemuri, B.C.: A Topology Independent Shape Modeling Scheme. Proc. SPIE Conf. on Geometric Methods in Computer Vision II **2031** (1993) 246–258, San Diego.

17. Malladi, R., Sethian, J.A., Vemuri, B.C.: Evolutionary Fronts for Topology-Independent Shape Modeling and Recovery. Proc. of the Third European Conference on Computer Vision, LNCS **800** (1994) 3–13, Stockholm, Sweden.

18. Malladi, R., Sethian, J.A., Vemuri, B.C.: Shape Modeling with Front Propagation: A Level Set Approach. IEEE Transactions on Pattern Analysis and Machine Intelligence. **17/2** (1995) 158–175.

19. March, R.: Visual Reconstruction with discontinuities using variational methods. Image and Vision Computing **10** (1992) 30–38.

20. Morel J.M., Solimini, S.: Variational Methods in Image Segmentation. Birkhäuser, PNLDE **14** (1994).

21. Mumford, D., Shah, J.: Optimal approximation by piecewise smooth functions and associated variational problems. Comm. Pure Appl. Math. **42** (1989) 577–685.

22. Osher, S., Sethian, J.A.: Fronts Propagating with Curvature-Dependent Speed: Algorithms Based on Hamilton-Jacobi Formulation. Journal of Computational Physics **79** (1988) 12–49.

23. Samson, C., Blanc-Féraud, L., Aubert, G., Zerubia, J.: A Level Set Model for Image Classification. M. Nilsen et al. (Eds.): Scale-Space'99, LNCS **1682** (1999) 306–317, Springer-Verlag Berlin Heidelberg.

24. Sapiro, G., Kimmel, R., Caselles, V.: Measurements in medical images via geodesic deformable contours. Proc. SPIE-Vision Geometry IV, Vol. **2573** (1995), San Diego, California.

25. Shah, J.: A Common Framework for Curve Evolution, Segmentation and Anisotropic Diffusion. IEEE Conference on Computer Vision and Pattern Recognition (1996).

26. Shah, J.: Riemannian Drums, Anisotropic Curve Evolution and Segmentation. M. Nilsen et al. (Eds.): Scale-Space'99, LNCS **1682** (1999) 129–140, Springer-Verlag Berlin Heidelberg.

27. Yezzi, A. Jr., Kichenassamy, S., Kumar, A., Olver, P., Tannenbaum, A.: A Geometric Snake Model for Segmentation of Medical Imagery. IEEE Transactions on Medical Imaging. **16/2** (1997) 199–209.

28. Yezzi, A., Tsai, A., Willsky, A.: A statistical approach to snakes for bimodal and trimodal imagery. Int. Conf. on Computer Vision (1999).

29. Zhao, H.-K., Chan, T., Merriman, B., Osher, S.: A Variational Level Set Approach to Multiphase Motion. J. Comput. Phys. **127** (1996) 179–195.

30. Zhu, S.C., Lee, T.S., Yuille, A.L.: Region competition: Unifying snakes, region growing, energy/Bayes/MDL for multi-band image segmentation. Proceedings of the IEEE 5th ICCV, Cambridge (1995) 416–423.

31. Zhu, S.C., Yuille, A.L.: Region competition: Unifying snakes, region growing, and Bayes/MDL for multi-band image segmentation. IEEE Transactions on Pattern Analysis and Machine Intelligence **18** (1996) 884–900.

5 Spherical Flattening of the Cortex Surface

A. Elad (Elbaz) and R. Kimmel

Technion–Israel Institute of Technology, Haifa 32000, Israel

Abstract. We present a novel technique to 'unfold' the curved convoluted outer surface of the brain known as the cortex and map it onto a sphere. The mapping procedure is constructed by first measuring the inter geodesic distances between points on the cortical surface. Next, a multi-dimensional scaling (MDS) technique is applied to map the whole or a section of the surface onto the sphere. The geodesic distances on the cortex are measured by the 'fast marching on triangulated domains' algorithm. It calculates the geodesic distances from a vertex on a triangulated surface to the rest of the vertices in $O(n)$ operations, where n is the number of vertices that represent the surface. Using this procedure, a matrix of the geodesic distances between every two vertices on the surface is computed. Next, a constrained MDS procedure finds the coordinates of points on a sphere such that the inter geodesic distances between points on the sphere are as close as possible to the geodesic distances measured between the corresponding points on the cortex. Thereby, our approach maximizes the goodness of fit of distances on the cortex surface to distances on the sphere. We apply our algorithm to sections of the human cortex, which is an extremely complex folded surface.

5.1 Introduction

The ability to compare between various cortical surfaces of either the same subject at different times, or cortex surfaces of different subjects, is essential in brain research. In order to achieve this goal it is vital to have a common and simple coordinate system that preserves the geometric structure of the cortical surface as much as possible. The rapid growth of the functional magnetic resonance imaging (fMRI) has motivated the development of new methods for analyzing and visualizing this neuroimaging data. One representation of fMRI data is by coloring the three-dimensional brain followed by volumetric rendering. However, this representation is difficult to visualize and analyze since most of the cortical surface is buried within sulci whose shape varies across individuals and whose form is quite complex. The ability to unfold and flatten the curved and convoluted outer surface of the brain onto a plane, or other simple surfaces that could serve as a unified coordinate system, would make the visualization and analysis of the cortex surface a much easier task.

A number of techniques have been proposed to obtain a flattened representation of the cortical surface. Few techniques flatten the surface onto a plane by preserving, as much as possible, the local distances between nodes on the given surface. While it is beyond the scope of this work to mention all the flattening methods, we briefly review the most related approaches. Schwartz,

Shaw, and Wolfson [13] were the first to apply MDS to a matrix of distances between neighboring nodes in a polyhedral representation of the surface, in order to select corresponding points in a plane that provide best fit in the least-square sense. The surface distances between nodes (up to eight nodes away form each other) were calculated using the method in [5], which involves in an exponential complexity procedure for the distance computation. This technique provides an optimal quasi-isometric mapping of the surface onto the plane.

Wandell at al. [16], flatten the cortical surface using a similar approach that constructs a 2D mesh that preserves the graph-geodesic distances between nodes on the cortical surface. A related approach, based on classical scaling and an improved graph-geodesic distances, was later proposed by Grossman et al. in [6]. Zigelman et al. [18] also applied classical MDS to a distances matrix between all vertices on a given surface. However, they used the numerically consistent *fast marching method on triangulated domains* [8] to calculate the geodesic distance between each pair of points. These techniques are the first to utilize the local as well as global distances between points on the given surface.

A conformal mapping for flattening was first introduced by Schwartz in [17], and later by Tannenbaum at al. [1]. The idea is to map a surface onto a disk or a sphere in a way that perseveres local angles. Recently, Haker at al. [7] used this method for texture mapping. This method preserves the metric 'locally', up to a local scale factor. It is based on the fact that the flattening function may be obtained as a solution of a second-ordered elliptic partial differential equation on the surface to be flattened. Although, in principle such a mapping is uniquely defined by the data, the local scaling deformations are sensitive to the data and the boundary conditions, and can serve as a coordinate frame of reference only for very special artificial cases.

In this paper, motivated by the above methods, we propose a novel technique to map sections of the cortex onto sections of a sphere by preserving local and global geodesic distances between points on the cortical surface. We solve the mapmaker's problem of mapping curved surfaces onto a sphere. The proposed method is based on two numerical procedures. The first, is the *fast marching on triangulated domains* [8], that efficiently calculates geodesic distances on triangulated curved surfaces. The second, is the Multi-Dimensional Scaling (MDS) [4,2,11], that uncovers the geometric structure of a set of data items from a (dis)similarity information among them. Mapping a curved surface onto a sphere is in general more complex than mapping onto a plane. Yet, for some surfaces like the cortex, that originally evolved from a sphere-like shape, the sphere serves as a more accurate coordinate system than the plane. Consequently, for curved surfaces such as section of the cortex, the mapping error to the plane is larger than the error of mapping onto a sphere, as illustrated in Fig. 5.1. Furthermore, since a finite plane can be considered as a small section of a sphere with infinite radius, our approach yields the same results obtained by planar flattening, in cases where the given surface is a plane like shape. For plane flattening we used a variation on Schwartz at al. [13] approach that handles both local and global geodesic distances computed by the fast marching method [8]. This method is the optimal flattening technique onto a plane that preserves the local as well as the global geodesic distances.

The outline of this paper is as follows: Section 2 gives brief review of the fast marching on triangulated domains algorithm. Section 3 presents the basic concepts of MDS and a detailed description of solving constrained MDS. Section 4 explains how these methods can be used to unfold curved surfaces onto a sphere. We conclude with future research directions in Section 5.

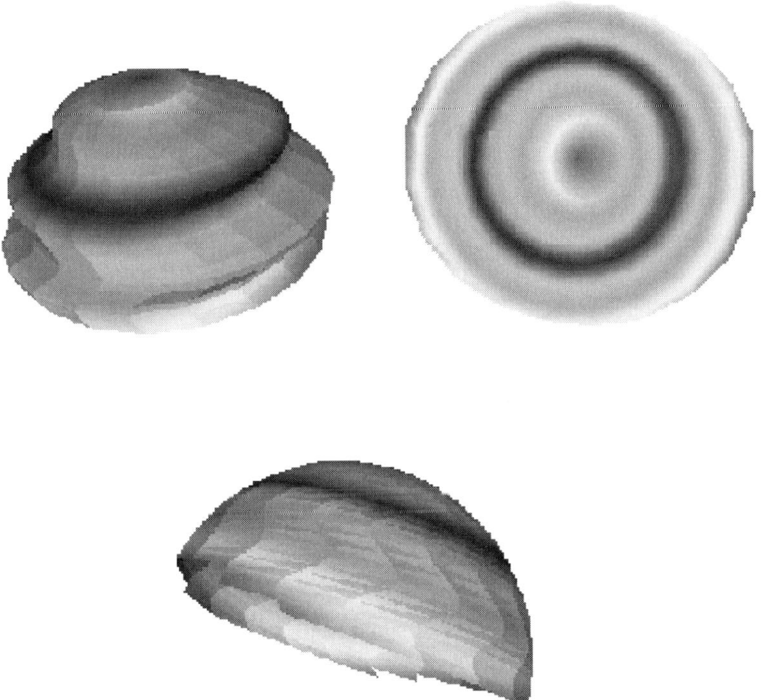

Fig. 5.1. Comparison between different flattening approaches. **Top left:** Original sphere-like surface. **Top right:** Planar flattening with matching error (Stress) = 0.0132. **Bottom:** Mapping onto a sphere with matching error (Stress) = 0.00945

5.2 Fast Marching Method on Triangulated Domains

The first step of our flattening procedure is finding the geodesic distances between pairs of points on the surface. The *fast marching method*, introduced by Sethian [14], is a numerical algorithm based on upwind finite difference approximations for solving the Eikonal equation; an equally fast technique for solving the Eikonal equation is due to Tsitsiklis [15], who makes use of Bellman's optimality criterion. It was extended to triangulated domains by Kimmel and Sethian in [8].

The basic idea is an efficient numerical approach that solves an Eikonal equation (defined by $|\nabla u| = 1$), where at the source point s the distance is known to be zero ($u(s) = 0$). For a specific choice of the numerical approximation, which is based on a monotone update scheme that is proven to converge to the 'viscosity' smooth solution, the solution u is the desired distance function. The idea is to iteratively construct the distance function by patching together small planes supported by neighboring grid points with gradient magnitude that equals to one. The distance function is constructed by starting from the sources point and propagating outwards. Applying the method to triangulated domains requires a careful analysis of the update of one vertex in a triangle, while the u values at the other vertices are given. For further details we refer to [8].

The fast marching method on triangulated domains can compute the geodesic distances between one vertex and the rest of the n surface vertices in $O(n)$ operations. Repeating this computation for each vertex, we compute a geodesic distances matrix D in $O(n^2)$ operations. Each ij entry of D represents the geodesic distance between the vertex i and the vertex j, that is

$$\delta_{ij} = \text{GeodesicDistance}(\text{Vertex}_i, \text{Vertex}_j)$$
$$[D]_{ij} = \delta_{ij}.$$

In order to reduce the computational effort, we sub-sample the surface vertices using the mesh-reduction technique proposed in [12]. Thereby, given a triangulated surface, we apply the fast marching procedure for each vertex in a representative set of the vertices as a source point, and obtain the geodesic distance matrix, D.

5.3 Multi-Dimensional Scaling

Multi-Dimensional Scaling (MDS) is a family of methods that map measurements of similarity or dissimilarity among pairs of feature items, into distances between feature points with given coordinates in a small-dimensional flat Euclidean space. The graphical display of the dissimilarity measurements, provided by MDS enables the analyst to 'look' at the data and explore its geometric structure visually. For example, given a set of feature items with proximity values among themselves, one can use MDS to construct a 2D flat map of these items, that is easier to comprehend and analyze. Most metrical MDS methods expect a set of n items and their pairwise (dis)similarities, and the desirable dimensionality, m, of the Euclidean embedding space.

The algorithm maps each item to a point x_i in an m dimensional Euclidean space $\Re^m$ by minimization of, for example, the stress function

$$S = \left(\frac{\sum_{i<j}(\delta_{ij} - d_{ij})^2}{\sum_{i<j} d_{ij}^2} \right)^{\frac{1}{2}}, \tag{5.1}$$

where δ_{ij} is the input dissimilarity measure between item i and j, d_{ij} is the Euclidean distance between these items in the m-dimensional Euclidean space. Here, we use as proximity values the geodesic distances between points on the given surface.

In some cases constraints are imposed on the configuration obtained from an MDS analysis, either through parameters or directly on the distances measured in the resulting configuration.

Cox and Cox [3] show how a configuration of points can be forced to lie on a surface of a sphere, based on a classic MDS method of Kruskal [10,9]. Let the points within a configuration on a sphere have spherical coordinates $(1, \theta_{i1}, \theta_{i2})$, $i = 1, 2...n$. In a Cartesian system these coordinates are

$$\begin{aligned} x_i &= \cos\theta_{i1}\sin\theta_{i2} \quad &-\frac{\pi}{2} \leq \theta_{i1} \leq \frac{\pi}{2} \\ y_i &= \sin\theta_{i1}\sin\theta_{i2} \\ z_i &= \cos\theta_{i2} \quad &0 \leq \theta_{i2} \leq 2\pi. \end{aligned} \tag{5.2}$$

The distance between two points is defined by the shortest arc-length measured along the great circle that passes through the points. This distance is proportional to the spherical angle between these points (the angle measured at the center of the sphere of radius R), and it is given by using the *cosine law*,

$$\varphi = \arccos\frac{2R^2 - (d_{ij}^e)^2}{2R^2}, \tag{5.3}$$

where d_{ij}^e is the Euclidean distance given by

$$d_{ij}^e = \left((x_i - x_j)^2 + (y_i - y_j)^2 + (z_i - z_j)^2\right)^{\frac{1}{2}}. \tag{5.4}$$

Using (5.2) we get that

$$d_{ij}^e = (2 - 2\sin\theta_{i2}\sin\theta_{j2}\cos(\theta_{i1} - \theta_{j1}) - 2\cos\theta_{i2}\cos\theta_{j2})^{\frac{1}{2}}. \tag{5.5}$$

We start with a set of random points, which lie on a sphere and iteratively update $(\boldsymbol{\theta}_1, \boldsymbol{\theta}_2)$ using the classic steepest-descent algorithm. The stress (5.1) can be written as

$$S = \left(\frac{S^*}{T^*}\right)^{\frac{1}{2}}$$

$$S^* = \sum_{i<j}(\delta_{ij} - d_{ij})^2$$

$$T^* = \sum_{i<j} d_{ij}^2. \tag{5.6}$$

The first derivatives of (5.6) is given by

$$\frac{\partial S}{\partial \theta_{lm}} = \frac{S}{2}\left(\frac{\partial S^*}{\partial \theta_{lm}} \cdot \frac{1}{S^*} - \frac{\partial T^*}{\partial \theta_{lm}} \cdot \frac{1}{T^*}\right) \quad l = 1, 2...n, \;\; m = 1, 2 \tag{5.7}$$

where

$$\frac{\partial S^*}{\partial \theta_{lm}} = 2\sum_{i=1}^{n}(d_{il} - \delta_{il})\frac{\partial d_{il}}{\partial \theta_{lm}}$$

$$\frac{\partial T^*}{\partial \theta_{lm}} = 2\sum_{i=1}^{n} d_{il}\frac{\partial d_{il}}{\partial \theta_{lm}}. \tag{5.8}$$

Cox and Cox [3] used the Euclidean distance instead of the arc-length itself and argued that there is a one to one increasing relationship between the Euclidean distance and the arc-length. Hence, setting $d_{ij} = d_{ij}^e$ and using (5.5), we get

$$\frac{\partial d_{il}}{\partial \theta_{l1}} = \frac{\partial d_{il}^e}{\partial \theta_{l1}} = \frac{1}{d_{il}^e}(-\sin\theta_{i2}\sin\theta_{l2}\sin(\theta_{i1} - \theta_{l1}))$$

$$\frac{\partial d_{il}}{\partial \theta_{l2}} = \frac{\partial d_{il}^e}{\partial \theta_{l2}} = \frac{1}{d_{il}^e}(-\sin\theta_{i2}\cos\theta_{l2}\cos(\theta_{i1} - \theta_{l1}) + \cos\theta_{i2}\sin\theta_{l2}). \tag{5.9}$$

Although this is a valid argument for using the Euclidean distances, it introduces some deformations on the configuration of the points. A simple example is mapping a section of a sphere onto a sphere. Specifically, consider the case where the given surface is half of a sphere embedded in a 3D Euclidean space $\Re^3$. Using the Euclidean distances instead of the geodesic distances on the sphere, we have that the distance between the farthest points is $2R$ instead of πR. Consequently, the configuration points after the mapping occupy a smaller section of the sphere as illustrated in Fig. 5.2.

Hence, for better accuracy, we use the arc length distance expression given in (5.3). Setting $d_{ij} = \varphi$, we have the first derivative of the arc-length distance, for $R = 1$, given by

$$\frac{\partial d_{il}}{\partial \theta_{lm}} = \frac{\partial \varphi}{\partial \theta_{lm}} = \frac{\partial d_{il}^e}{\partial \theta_{lm}} \cdot \frac{d_{il}^e}{\sqrt{1 - \left(\frac{2-(d_{il}^e)^2}{2}\right)^2}}. \tag{5.10}$$

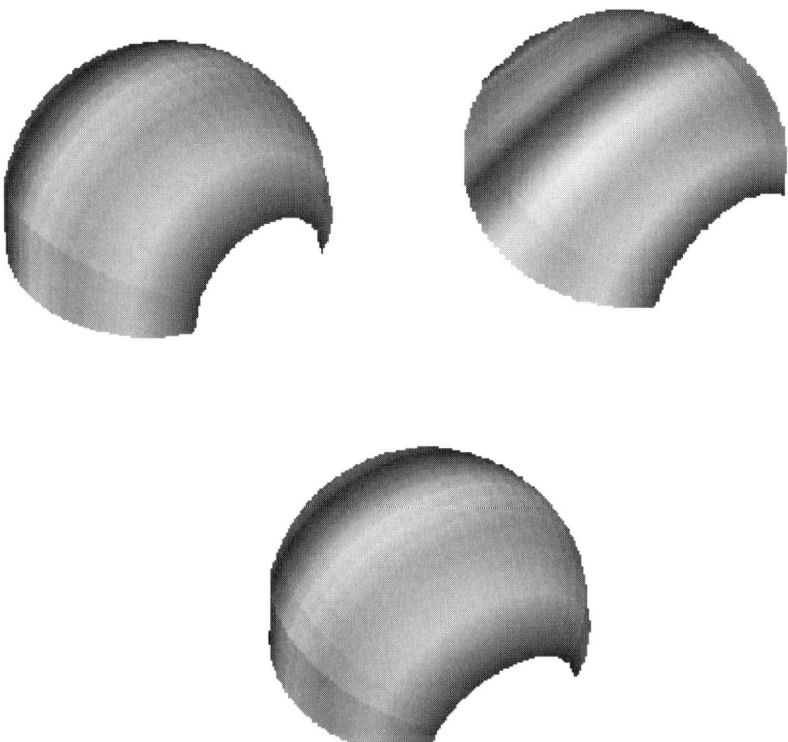

Fig. 5.2. Sphere flattening using Euclidean and arc-length distances. **Top left**: Original surface. **Top right:** Cox [3] approach using Euclidean distance. **Bottom:** Our approach using the arc-length geodesic distance on the target sphere

In order to avoid estimating the desired radius of the sphere, we normalized the distance matrices, $D = [\delta_{ij}]$ and $\hat{D} = [d_{ij}]$, so that instead of having the absolute distances we use the relative distance. This way, we fix R and the relative distances spread the points on the proper section of the sphere.

For illustration, Figures 5.3 and 5.4 show the results of mapping a planar surface and a human face onto a sphere. We notice that the stress error of flattening onto a plane is a bit higher as expected for the human face example. As stated above, for plane-like surfaces this approach converges to a spherical solution with an infinite radius. Hence, even for the open plane example, the planar flattening is a bit less accurate mainly due to the small numerical errors in the geodesic distance measurements.

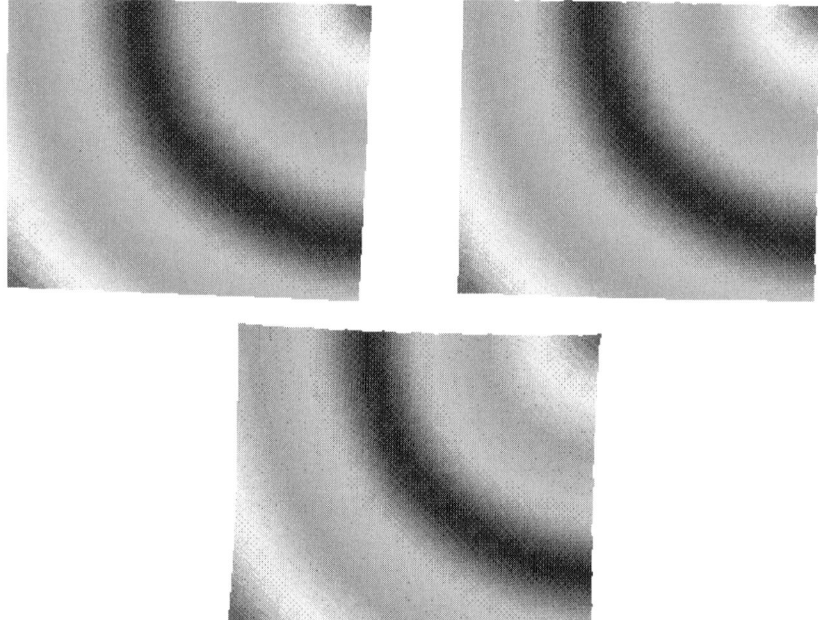

Fig. 5.3. Comparison between different flattening approaches for plane. **Top left:** Original surface. **Top right:** Planar flattening (Stress $=$ 0.0000312). **Bottom:** mapping onto a sphere (Stress $=$ 0.0000309)

5.4   Cortex Unfolding

Equipped with the fast marching on triangulated domains, and the constrained MDS on a sphere, we map a given section of cortical brain surface, represented by n vertices, onto a sphere. We take the following steps.

a. Construct the geodesic distances matrix, $D_{n \times n}$, by application of the fast marching procedure to each vertex.
b. Select a set of n randomly distributed points that lie on a sphere.
c. Calculate the distances matrix, $\hat{D}$, by using either the Euclidean distance (5.4) or the spherical geodesic stance (5.3).
d. Compute the stress (5.1) for the given configuration of the points.
e. If the stress error does not improve by more than a given threshold then STOP.
f. Calculate the first gradients of the stress function (5.1) according to (5.9) or (5.10).
g. Update $(\boldsymbol{\theta}_1, \boldsymbol{\theta}_2)$ in the conjugate gradient direction of the stress and compute the new configuration points.
h. Go to step c.

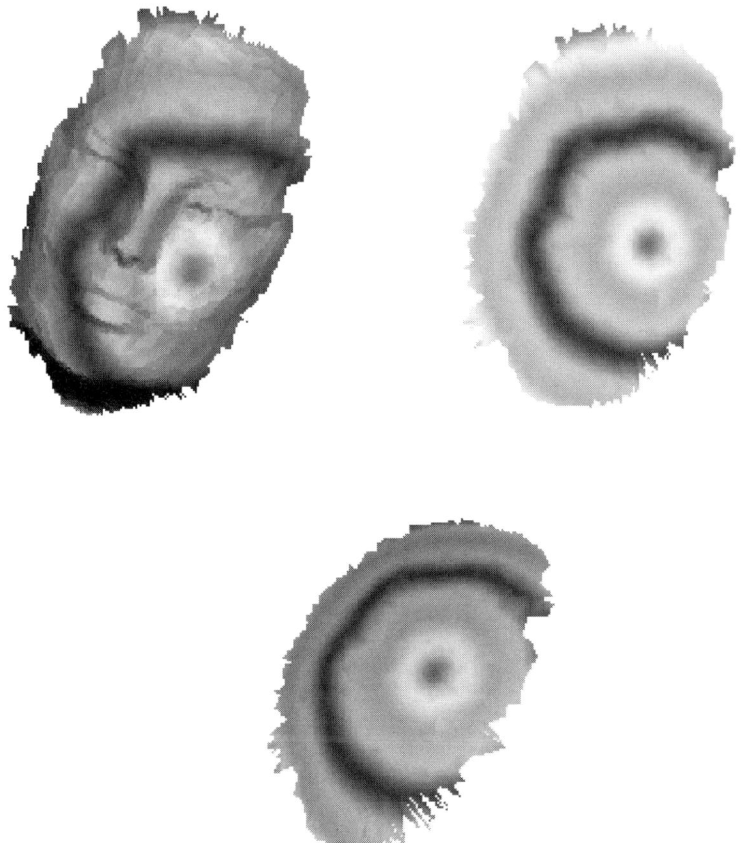

Fig. 5.4. Comparison between different flattening approaches for a human face. **Top left:** Original surface. **Top right:** Planar flattening (Stress = 0.000314). **Bottom:** mapping onto a sphere (Stress = 0.000312)

This procedure converges to the same stress independently of the initial configurations of the points. Since the stress (5.1) is a function of the interpoint distances, the solution is determined up to rotation and reflection.

In order to extract a practical algorithm from the above definitions we use the following approximation steps. First, we assume that the given triangulated surface of the cortex is a good approximation of the continuous one. Next, for the computational efficiency of the MDS-flattening step, we consider only a subset of the given vertices. These steps were verified empirically to introduce minor deformations in the results. The sub-sampling technique is an iterative process where in each iteration the farthest (in the geodesic sense) vertex from the already selected vertices is selected. The process starts by selecting the first vertex randomly, and terminates when the sub-set of selected vertices reaches a pre-defined number (in our examples 1000-5000 vertices).

Figures 5.5, 5.6 and 5.7 show the results of mapping different sections of the cortex onto a sphere. Planar flattening results are provided as well as the stress obtained by mapping onto a sphere instead of a plane. We notice that for relatively small portions of the brain (1000-10000 vertices) the planar and the spherical flattening approaches are quite close, while as the sections of the brain surfaces get larger (more than 10K vertices in our examples) the residual error is clearly better for the spherical mapping as argued above. To verify that the mapping preserves distances, we applied a simple texture mapping technique to the original surface and then mapped it to the configuration points obtained by the flattening procedure. The texture we used is based on coloring each vertex according to it's geodesic distance from a specific vertex. Using this texture we should have obtain concentric circles on the flattened surface as in Figs. 5.5, 5.6 and 5.7.

5.5   Conclusions

An efficient and accurate method for flattening sections of the cortex surface onto a sphere was presented. The method is based on the fast marching on triangulated domains algorithm followed by a special multi-dimensional scaling (MDS) technique. The flattening result onto a sphere is computed by applying a constrained MDS procedure on the geodesic distances matrix obtained by the fast marching algorithm. This is a numerical solution to the general mapmaker's problem onto a sphere. It was shown to give better results than planar flattening for large sections of the cortical surface.

References

1. S. Angenent, S. Haker, A. Tannenbaum, and R. Kikinis. On the laplace-beltrami operator and brain surface flattening. *IEEE Trans. on Medical Imaging*, 18(8):700–711, August 1999.
2. I. Borg and P. Groenen. *Modern Multidimensional Scaling - Theory and Applications*. Springer, 1997.
3. M. Cox and T. Cox. Multidimensional scaling on a sphere. *Commun. Statist*, 20(9):2943–2953, 1991.
4. M. Cox and T. Cox. *Multidimensional Scaling*. Chapman and Hall, 1994.
5. C. Frederick and E. L. Schwartz. Confromal image warping. *IEEE Trans. Pattern Anal. Machine Intell*, 11(9):1005–1008, 1989.
6. R. Grossman, N. Kiryati, and R. Kimmel. Computational surface flattening: A voxel-based approach. , *Lecture Notes in Computer Science*, 2059:196–204, 2001.

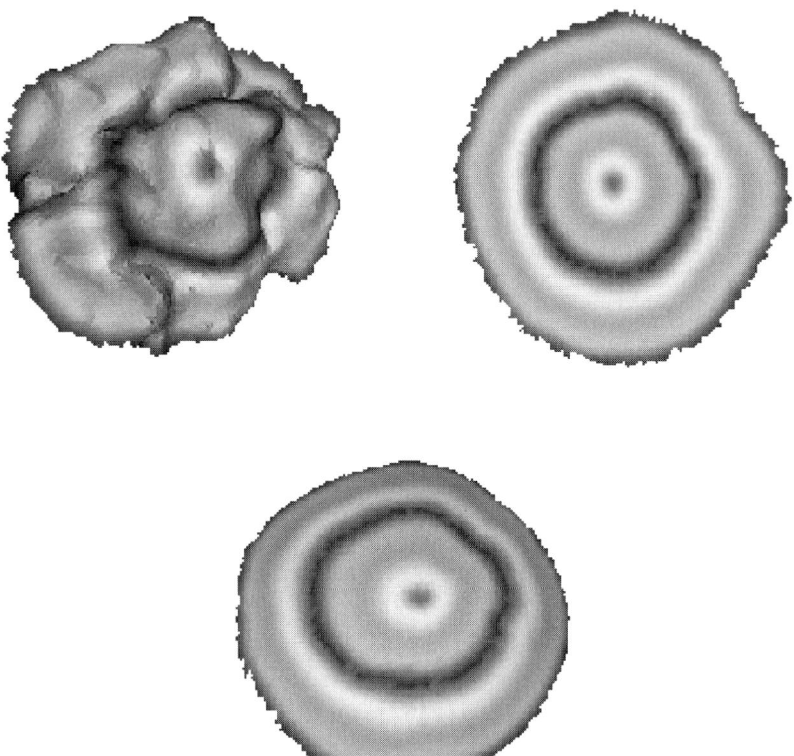

Fig. 5.5. Flattening a section of a human cortex. **Top left:** Original surface (3000 vertices). **Top right:** Planar flattening (Stress = 0.0020). **Bottom:** Mapping onto a sphere (Stress = 0.0011)

7. S. Haker, S. Angenent, A. Tannenbaum, R. Kikinis, G. Sapiro, and M. Halle. Conformal surface parameterization for texture mapping. *IEEE Trans. on Visualization and Computer Graphics*, 6:181–189, 2000.

8. R. Kimmel and J. Sethian. Computing geodesic on manifolds. *Proc. of National Academy of Science*, 95:8431–8435, 1998.

9. J. Kruskal. Multidimensional scaling: anumerical method. *Psychometrika*, 36:57–62, 1964.

10. J. Kruskal. Multidimensional scaling by optimizinggoodness of-fit to a non-metric hypothesis. *Psychometrika*, 29:1–27, 1964.

11. J. B. Kruskal and M. Wish. *Multidimensional Scaling*. Sage, 1978.

12. S. Melax. A simple, fast and effective polygon reduction algorithm. *Game Developer Journal*, November 1998.

13. E. L. Schwartz, A. Shaw, and E. Wolfson. A numerical solution to the generalized mapmaker's problem: Flattening nonconvex polyhedral surfaces. *IEEE Trans. Pattern Anal. Machine Intell*, 11(9):1005–1008, 1989.

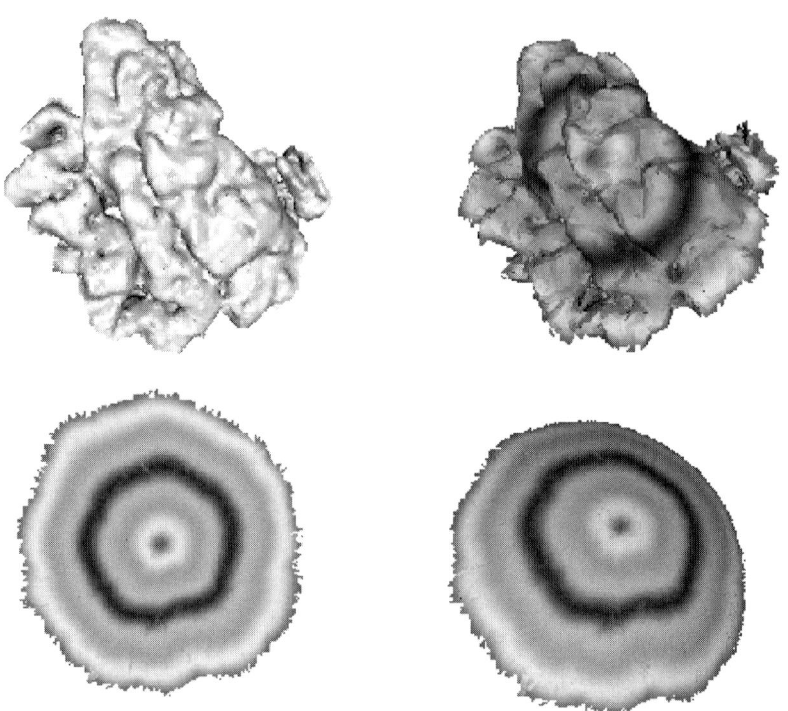

Fig. 5.6. Flattening a section of a human cortex. **Top left:** Original surface (20000 vertices). **Top right:** Decimated surface (5000 vertices). **Bottom left:** Planar flattening (Stress = 0.0038). **Bottom right:** Mapping onto a sphere (Stress = 0.0022)

14. J. Sethian. A review of the theory, algorithms, and applications of level set method for propagating surfaces. *Acta Numerica, Cambridge University Press*, 1996.

15. J. N. Tsitsiklis. Efficient algorithms for globally optimal trajectories. *IEEE Trans. on Automatic Control*, 40:1528–1538, 1995.

16. B. A. Wandell, S. Chial, and B. Backus. Visualization and measurements of the cortical surface. *Journal of Cognitive Neuroscience*, January 2000.

17. E. Wolfson and E. L. Schwartz. Computing minimal distances on arbitrary two-dimensional polyhedral surfaces. *IEEE Computer Graphics and Applications*, 1990.

18. G. Zigelman and R. Kimmel. Texture mapping using surface flattening via MDS. *Accepted to IEEE Trans. on Visualization and Computer Graphics*, 2001.

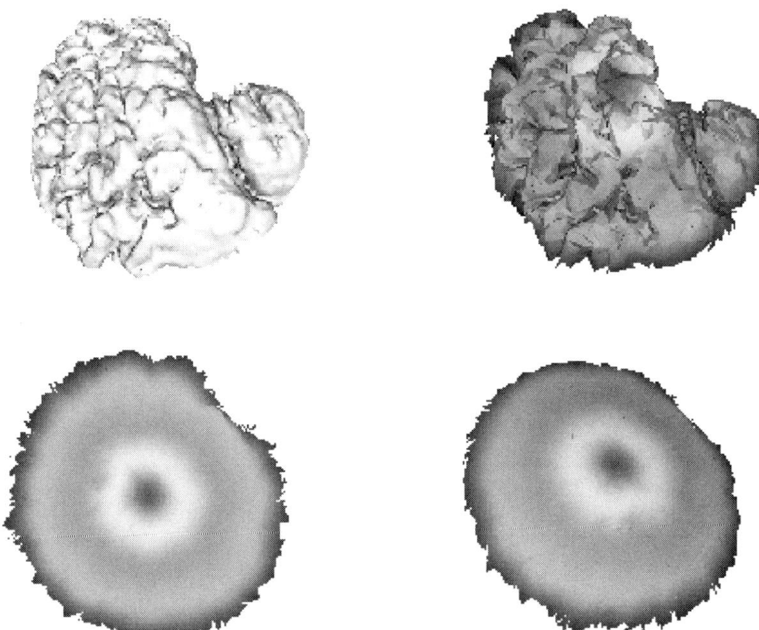

Fig. 5.7. Flattening a section of a human cortex. **Top left:** Original surface (56000 vertices). **Top right:** Decimated surface (3500 vertices). **Bottom left:**Planar flattening (Stress = 0.0088). **Bottom right:** Mapping onto a sphere (Stress = 0.0060)

6 Grouping Connected Components using Minimal Path Techniques

T. Deschamps[1,2] and L. D. Cohen[2]

[1] Medical Imaging Systems Group, Philips Research France,
51 rue Carnot, 92156 Suresnes, France
Email: thomas.deschamps@philips.com
[2] Laboratoire CEREMADE, UMR 7534, Université Paris Dauphine,
75775 Paris cedex 16, France,
Email: cohen@ceremade.dauphine.fr

Abstract. We address the problem of finding a set of contour curves in a 2D or 3D image. We consider the problem of perceptual grouping and contour completion, where the data is an unstructured set of regions in the image. A new method to find complete curves from a set of edge points is presented. Contours are found as minimal paths between connected components, using the fast marching algorithm. We find the minimal paths between each of these components, until the complete set of these "regions" is connected. The paths are obtained using backpropagation from the saddle points to both components.

We then extend this technique to 3D. The data is a set of connected components in a 3D image. We find 3D minimal paths that link together these components. Using a potential based on vessel detection, we illustrate the capability of our approach to reconstruct tree structures in a 3D medical image dataset.

6.1 Introduction

We are interested in perceptual grouping and finding a set of curves in an image with the use of energy minimizing curves. Since their introduction, active contours [10] have been extensively used to find the contour of an object in an image through the minimization of an energy. In order to get a set of contours with T-junctions, we need many active contours to be initialized on the image. The level sets paradigm [13,1] allowed changes in topology. It enables to get multiple contours by starting with a single one. However, these do not give satisfying results when there are gaps in the data since the contour may propagate into a hole and then split to many curves where only one contour is desired. This is the problem encountered with perceptual grouping where a set of incomplete contours is given. For example, in a binary image like in figure 6.1 with a drawing of a shape with holes, human vision can easily fill in the missing boundaries and form complete curves. Perceptual grouping is an old problem in computer vision. It has been approached more recently with energy methods [15,9,16]. These methods find a criteria for saliency of a curve component or for each point of the image. In these methods, the definition of saliency measure is based indirectly on a second order regularization snake-like energy ([10]) of a path containing the point. However, the final curves are obtained generally in a second step as ridge lines of the saliency criteria after thresholding. Motivated by this relation between energy minimizing curves like snakes and completion contours, we are interested in finding a set of completion contours on an image as a set of energy minimizing curves.

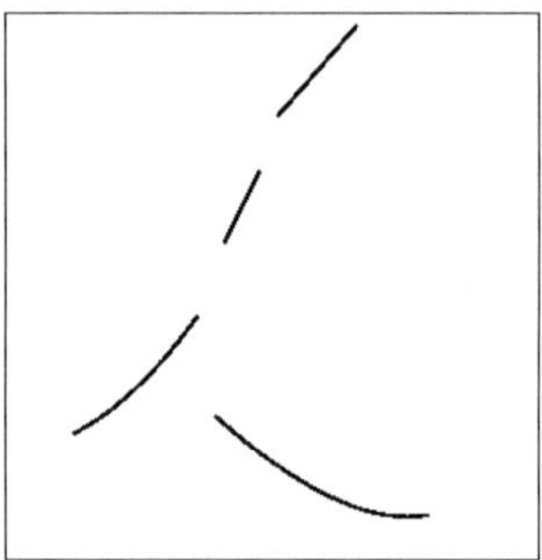

Fig. 6.1. Examples of connected regions to be completed

In order to solve global minimization for snakes, the authors of [4] used the minimal paths, as introduced in [12,11]. The goal was to avoid local minima without demanding too much on user initialization, which is a main drawback of classic snakes [2]. Only two end points were needed. The numerical method has the advantage of being consistent (see [4]) and efficient using the Fast Marching algorithm introduced in [14].

In [3], we proposed a way to use this minimal path approach to find a set of curves drawn from a set of points in the image. We also introduced a technique that automatically finds a set of *key* end points. In this paper, we extend the previous approach to connected components instead of end points. In order to obtain a set of most salient contour curves, we find a set of minimal paths between pairs of connected components.

This approach is then extended for application in the completion of tube-like structures in 2D and 3D images. The problem is here to complete a partially detected object, based on some detected connected components that belong to this object.

For perceptual grouping, the potential P to be minimized along the curves is usually an image of edge points that represent simple incomplete shapes, as in figure 6.1. These edge points are represented as a binary image with small potential values along the edges and high values at the background. The potential could also be defined as edges weighted by the value of the gradient or as a function of an estimate of the gradient of the image itself, $P = g(\|\nabla I\|)$, like in classic snakes. The potential could also be a grey level image as in [4]. It could also be a more complicated function of the grey level.

In our real examples of vascular structures in 2D and 3D, we use a potential based on a vesselness filter [8].

The paper is presented as follows. We first give a summary of minimal paths and fast marching in 2D and 3D images in section 6.2. We then present in Section 6.3 how to find a set of curves from a given set of unstructured points. Grouping the points in connected components, we propose a way to find the pairs of linked connected components and the paths between them. We then extend this approach to 3D and show an application in 3D medical images.

6.2   Minimal Paths in 2D and 3D

6.2.1   Global Minimum for Active Contours

We present in this section the basic ideas of the method introduced in [4] to find the global minimum of the active contour energy using minimal paths. The energy to minimize is similar to classical deformable models (see [10]) where it combines smoothing terms and image features attraction term (Potential P):

$$E(C) = \int_{\Omega} \left\{ w_1 \|C'(s)\|^2 + w_2 \|C''(s)\|^2 + P(C(s)) \right\} ds \qquad (6.1)$$

where $C(s)$ represents a curve drawn on a 2D image and Ω is its domain of definition. The authors of [4] have related this problem with the recently introduced paradigm of the level-set formulation. In particular, its Euler equation is equivalent to the geodesic active contours [1]. The method introduced in [4] improves energy minimization because the problem is transformed in a way to find the global minimum.

6.2.2   Problem formulation

As explained in [4], we are lead to minimize

$$E(C) = \int_{\Omega=[0,L]} \{w + P(C(s))\} ds, \qquad (6.2)$$

where s is the arclength parameter ($\|C'(s)\| = 1$). The regularization of this model is now achieved by the constant $w > 0$ (see [4] for details). Given a potential $P \geq 0$, the energy is like a distance weighted by $\tilde{P} = P + w$. The minimal action $\mathcal{U}$ is defined as the minimal energy integrated along a path between a starting point p_0 and any point p:

$$\mathcal{U}(p) = \inf_{\mathcal{A}_{p_0,p}} E(C) = \inf_{\mathcal{A}_{p_0,p}} \left\{ \int_{\Omega} P(C(s)) ds \right\} \qquad (6.3)$$

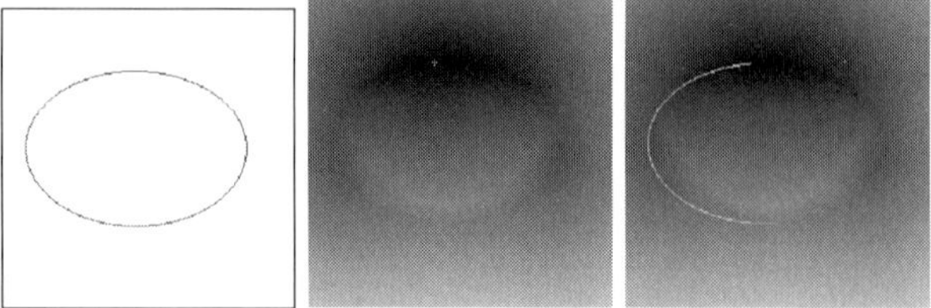

Fig. 6.2. Finding a minimal path between two points. On the left, the potential is minimal on the ellipse. In the middle, the minimal action or weighted distance to the marked point. On the right, minimal path using backpropagation from the second point.

where $\mathcal{A}_{p_0,p}$ is the set of all paths between p_0 and p. The minimal path between p_0 and any point p_1 in the image can be easily deduced from this action map by a simple back-propagation (gradient descent on $\mathcal{U}$) starting from p_1 until p_0 is reached.

6.2.3   Fast Marching Resolution

In order to compute this map $\mathcal{U}$, a front-propagation equation related to Equation (6.3) is solved:

$$\frac{\partial C}{\partial t} = \frac{1}{\tilde{P}}\overrightarrow{n}. \tag{6.4}$$

It evolves a front starting from an infinitesimal circle shape around p_0 until each point inside the image domain is assigned a value for $\mathcal{U}$. The value of $\mathcal{U}(p)$ is the time t at which the front passes over the point p.

The *Fast Marching* technique, introduced in [14], was used in [4] noticing that the map $\mathcal{U}$ satisfies the Eikonal equation:

$$\|\nabla \mathcal{U}\| = \tilde{P} \quad \text{and} \quad \mathcal{U}(p_0) = 0. \tag{6.5}$$

Classic finite differences schemes for this equation tend to overshoot and are unstable. An up-wind scheme was proposed by [14]. It relies on a one-sided derivative that looks in the up-wind direction of the moving front, and thereby avoids the over-shooting associated with finite differences:

$$(\max\{u - \mathcal{U}_{i-1,j}, u - \mathcal{U}_{i+1,j}, 0\})^2 +$$
$$(\max\{u - \mathcal{U}_{i,j-1}, u - \mathcal{U}_{i,j+1}, 0\})^2 = \tilde{P}_{i,j}^2, \tag{6.6}$$

giving the correct viscosity-solution u for $\mathcal{U}_{i,j}$. The improvement made by the *Fast Marching* is to introduce order in the selection of the grid points. This order is based on the fact that information is propagating *outward*, because the action can only grow due to the quadratic Equation (6.6).

This technique of considering at each step only the necessary set of grid points was originally introduced for the construction of minimum length paths

Algorithm for 2D Fast Marching

- Definitions:
    - *Alive* set: grid points at which the action value $\mathcal{U}$ has been reached and will not be changed;
    - *Trial* set: next grid points (4-connexity neighbors) to be examined. An estimate U of $\mathcal{U}$ has been computed using Eqn. (6.6) from alive points only (i.e. from $\mathcal{U}$);
    - *Far* set: all other grid points, there is not yet an estimate for U;
- Initialization:
    - *Alive* set: start point p_0, $U(p_0) = \mathcal{U}(p_0) = 0$;
    - *Trial* set: reduced to the four neighbors p of p_0 with initial value $U(p) = \tilde{P}(p)$ $(\mathcal{U}(p) = \infty)$;
    - *Far* set: all other grid points, $\mathcal{U} = U = \infty$;
- Loop:
    - Let $p = (i_{min}, j_{min})$ be the *Trial* point with the smallest action U;
    - Move it from the *Trial* to the *Alive* set;
    - For each neighbor (i, j) of (i_{min}, j_{min}):
        * If (i, j) is *Far*, add it to the *Trial* set;
        * If (i, j) is *Trial*, update $U_{i,j}$ with Eqn. (6.6).

Table 6.1. *Fast Marching* algorithm

in a graph between two given nodes in [7]. The algorithm is detailed in Table 6.1. An example is shown in Figure 6.2. The *Fast Marching* technique selects at each iteration the *Trial* point with minimum action value. In order to compute this value, we have to solve Equation (6.7) for each trial point, as detailed in section 6.2.4.

6.2.4 Algorithm for 2D Up-Wind Scheme

Notice that for solving Eqn. (6.6), only alive points are considered. Considering the neighbors of grid point (i, j) in 4-connexity, we note $\{A_1, A_2\}$ and $\{B_1, B_2\}$ the two couples of opposite neighbors such that we get the ordering $\mathcal{U}(A_1) \leq \mathcal{U}(A_2)$, $\mathcal{U}(B_1) \leq \mathcal{U}(B_2)$, and $\mathcal{U}(A_1) \leq \mathcal{U}(B_1)$. Considering that we have $u \geq \mathcal{U}(B_1) \geq \mathcal{U}(A_1)$, the equation derived is

$$(u - \mathcal{U}(A_1))^2 + (u - \mathcal{U}(B_1))^2 = \tilde{P}_{i,j}^2 \tag{6.7}$$

Based on testing the discriminant Δ of Eqn. (6.7), one or two neighbors are used to solve it:

1. If $\tilde{P}_{i,j} > \mathcal{U}(B_1) - \mathcal{U}(A_1)$, solution of Eqn. (6.7) is
$$u = \frac{\mathcal{U}(B_1) + \mathcal{U}(A_1) + \sqrt{2\tilde{P}_{i,j}^2 - (\mathcal{U}(B_1) - \mathcal{U}(A_1))^2}}{2}.$$
2. else $u = \mathcal{U}(A_1) + \tilde{P}_{i,j}$.

6.2.5 Minimal Paths in 3D

A 3D extension of the *Fast Marching* algorithm was presented in [5] and detailed in [6]. Similarly to previous section, the minimal action $\mathcal{U}$ is defined as

$$\mathcal{U}(p) = \inf_{\mathcal{A}_{p_0,p}} \left\{ \int_\Omega \tilde{P}(C(s))ds \right\} \tag{6.8}$$

where $\mathcal{A}_{p_0,p}$ is now the set of all 3D paths between p_0 and p. Given a start point p_0, in order to compute $\mathcal{U}$ we start from an initial infinitesimal front around p_0. The 2D scheme equation (6.6) is extended to 3D, leading to the scheme

$$\begin{aligned}
(\max\{u - \mathcal{U}_{i-1,j,k}, u - \mathcal{U}_{i+1,j,k}, 0\})^2 \; + \\
(\max\{u - \mathcal{U}_{i,j-1,k}, u - \mathcal{U}_{i,j+1,k}, 0\})^2 \; + \\
(\max\{u - \mathcal{U}_{i,j,k-1}, u - \mathcal{U}_{i,j,k+1}, 0\})^2 = \tilde{P}^2_{i,j,k}
\end{aligned} \tag{6.9}$$

giving the correct viscosity-solution u for $\mathcal{U}_{i,j,k}$.

6.3   Finding Contours from a Set of Connected Components R_k

6.3.1   Minimal Path between two Regions

The method of [4], detailed in the previous section allows to find a minimal path between two endpoints. This is a straightforward extension to define a minimal path between two regions of the image. Given two connected regions of the image R_0 and R_1, we consider R_0 as the starting region and R_1 as a set of end points. The problem is then finding a path minimizing energy among all paths with start point in R_0 and end point in R_1. The minimal action is now defined by

$$\mathcal{U}(p) = \inf_{\mathcal{A}_{R_0,p}} E(C) = \inf_{p_0 \in R_0} \inf_{\mathcal{A}_{p_0,p}} E(C) \tag{6.10}$$

where $\mathcal{A}_{R_0,p}$ is the set of all paths starting at a point of R_0 and ending at p. This minimal action can be computed the same way as before in table 6.1, with the alive set initialized as the whole set of points of R_0, with $\mathcal{U} = 0$ and trial points being the set of 4-connexity neighbors of points of R_0 that are not in R_0. Backpropagation by gradient descent on $\mathcal{U}$ from any point p in the image will give the minimal path that join this point with region R_0.

In order to find a minimal path between region R_1 and region R_0, we determine a point $p_1 \in R_1$ such that $\mathcal{U}(p_1) = \min_{p \in R_1} \mathcal{U}(p)$. We then backpropagate from p_1 to R_0 to find the minimal path between p_1 and R_0, which is also a minimal path between R_1 and R_0.

6.3.2   Minimal Paths from a Set of Connected Components

We are now interested in finding many or all contours in an image. We assume that from some preprocessing, or as data, we have an initial set of contours.

We denote R_k the connected components of these contours. We propose to find the contours as a set of minimal paths that link pairs of regions among the R_k's. If we also know which pairs of regions have to be linked together, finding the whole set of contours is a trivial application of the previous section. The problem we are interested in here is also to find out which pairs of regions have to be connected by a contour. Since the set of contours R_k's is assumed to be given unstructured, we do not know in advance how the regions connect. This is the key problem that is solved here using a minimal action map.

6.3.3   Method

Our approach is similar to computing the distance map to a set of regions and their Voronoi diagram. However, we use here a weighted distance defined through the potential P. This distance is obtained as the minimal action with respect to P with zero value at all points of regions R_k. Instead of computing a minimal action map for each pair of regions, as in Section 6.3.1, we only need to compute one minimal action map in order to find all paths. At the same time the action map is computed we determine the pairs of regions that have to be linked together. This is based on finding meeting points of the propagation fronts. These are *saddle points* of the minimal action $\mathcal{U}$. In Section 6.2, we said that calculation of the minimal action can be seen as the propagation of a front through equation (6.4). Although the minimal action is computed using fast marching, the level sets of $\mathcal{U}$ give the evolution of the front. During the fast marching algorithm, the boundary of the set of alive points also gives the position of the front. In the previous section, we had only one front evolving from the starting region R_0. Since all points p of regions R_k are set with $\mathcal{U}(p) = 0$, we now have one front evolving from each of the starting regions R_k. In what follows when we talk about front meeting, we mean either the geometric point where the two fronts coming from different R_k's meet, or in the discrete algorithm the first alive point which connects two components from different R_k's (see Figures 6.3 and 6.4).

We use the fact that given two regions R_1 and R_2, the saddle point S where the two fronts starting from each region meet can be used to find the minimal path between R_1 and R_2. Indeed, the minimal path between the two regions has to pass by the meeting point S. This point is the point half way (in energy) on a minimal path between R_1 and R_2. Backpropagating from S to R_1 and then from S to R_2 gives the two halves of the path.

6.3.4   Notations and definitions

Here are some definitions that will be used in what follows. X being a set of points in the image, $\mathcal{U}_X$ is the minimal action obtained by Fast Marching with potential $\tilde{P}$ and starting points $\{p, p \in X\}$. This means that all points of X are initialized as alive points with value 0. All their 4-connexity neighbors

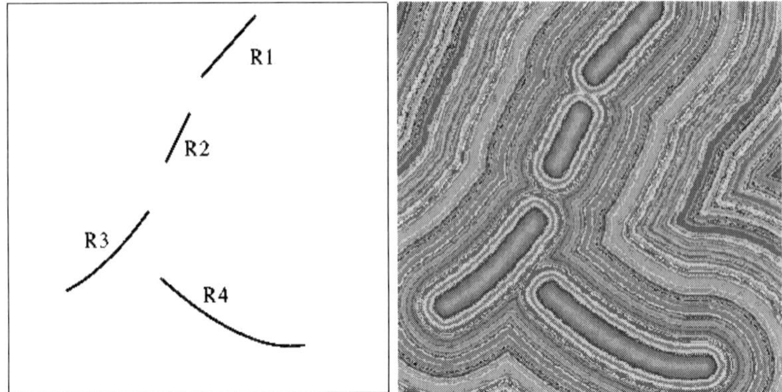

Fig. 6.3. Minimal Action map from the four regions of the example of figure 6.1. On the right with a random LUT to show the level sets.

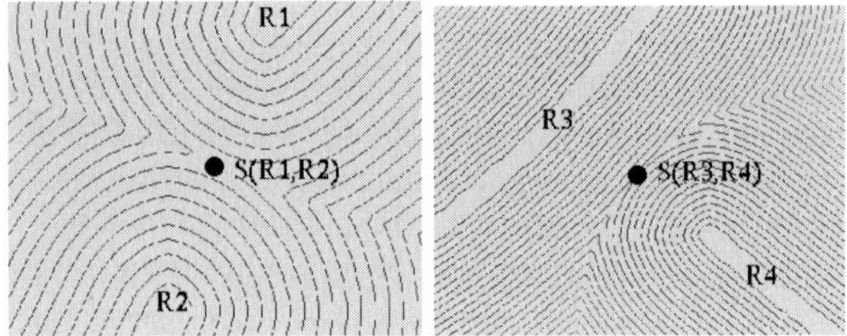

Fig. 6.4. Zoom on *saddle points* between regions.

that are not in X are *trial* points. This is easy to see that $\mathcal{U}_X = \min_{p \in X} \mathcal{U}_p$. X may be a connected component R or a set of connected components.

The *label* l at a point p is equal to the index k of the region R_k for p closer in energy to R_k than to other regions R_j. This means that minimal action $\mathcal{U}_{R_k}(p) \leq \mathcal{U}_{R_j}(p), \forall j \neq k$. We define the region $L_k = \{p/l(p) = k\}$. If $X = \cup_j R_j$, we have $\mathcal{U}_X = \mathcal{U}_{R_k}$ on L_k and the computation of $\mathcal{U}_X$ is the same as the simultaneous computation of each $\mathcal{U}_{R_k}$ on each region L_k. These are the simultaneous fronts starting from each R_k.

A *saddle point* $S(R_i, R_j)$ between R_i and R_j is the first point where the front starting from R_i to compute $\mathcal{U}_{R_i}$ meets the front starting from R_j to compute $\mathcal{U}_{R_j}$; At this point, $\mathcal{U}_{R_i}$ and $\mathcal{U}_{R_j}$ are equal and this is the smallest value for which they are equal.

Two different regions among the R_k's will be called *linked regions* if they are selected to be linked together. The way we choose to link two regions is to select some *saddle points*. Thus regions R_i and R_j are *linked regions* if their *saddle point* is among the selected ones.

A *cycle* is a sequence of different regions $R_k, 1 \leq k \leq K$, such that for $1 \leq k \leq K - 1$, R_k and R_{k+1} are *linked regions* and R_K and R_1 are also *linked regions*.

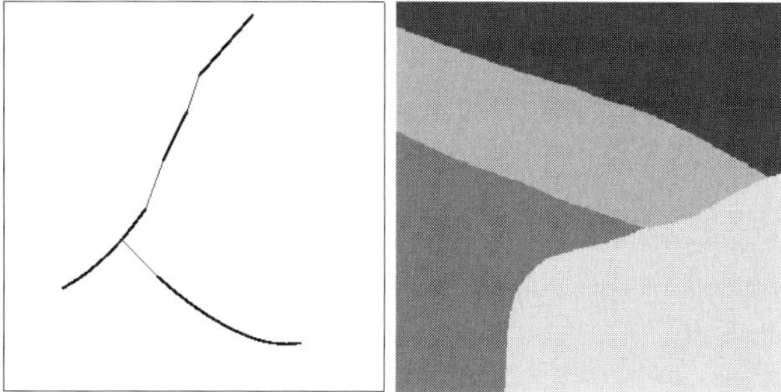

Fig. 6.5. Example with four regions. On the left we show the minimal paths obtained by backpropagation from the three *saddle points* to each of the regions from where the front comes; on the right, and the Voronoi diagram obtained.

6.3.5   Finding and Selecting Saddle Points

The main goal of our method is to obtain all significant paths joining the given regions. However, each region should not be connected to all other regions, but only to those that are closer to them in the energy sense. There are many possibilities for deciding which regions connect together depending on the kind of data and application. In some cases, the goal would be to detect closed curves and avoid forming branches, as in [3]. Then the criterion would be to constrain a region to be linked to at most two other regions in order to make *cycles*. In our context, we are interested in detecting branches and avoiding closed curves. Therefore the criterion for two regions R_i and R_j to be connected is that their fronts meet without creating a "cycle".

We see in Figure 6.4 a zoom on the saddle points detected between regions R_1 and R_2 and R_3 and R_4. Once a *saddle point* $S(R_i, R_j)$ is found and selected, backpropagation relatively to final energy $\mathcal{U}$ should be done both ways to R_i and to R_j to find the two halves of the path between them. We see in Figure 6.5 this backpropagation at each of the three automatically selected *saddle points*. They link R_1 to R_2, R_2 to R_3 and R_3 to R_4. At a saddle point, the gradient is zero, but the direction of descent towards each point are opposite. For each backpropagation, the direction of descent is the one relative to each region. This means that in order to estimate the gradient direction toward R_i, all points in a region different from L_i have their energy put artificially to ∞. This allows finding the good direction for the gradient descent towards R_i. However, as mentioned earlier, these backpropagations have to be done only for selected *saddle points*. In the fast marching algorithm we have a simple way to find *saddle points* and update the *linked regions*.

As defined above, the region L_k associated with a region R_k is the set of points p of the image such that minimal energy $\mathcal{U}_{R_k}(p)$ to R_k is smaller than all the $\mathcal{U}_{R_j}(p)$ to other regions R_j. The set of such regions L_k covers the whole image, and forms the Voronoi diagram of the image (see figure 6.5). All *saddle points* are at a boundary between two regions L_k. For a

---

Minimal paths between Regions R_k

- Initialization:
    - R_k's are given
    - $\forall k, \forall p \in R_k, V(p) = 0; l(p) = k;\ p$ *alive*.
    - $\forall p \notin \cup_k R_k, V(p) = \infty; l(p) = -1;\ p$ is *far* except 4-connexity neighbors of R_k's that are *trial* with estimate U using Eqn. 6.6.
- Loop for computing $V = \mathcal{U}_{\cup_k R_k}$:
    - Let $p = (i_{min}, j_{min})$ be the *Trial* point with the smallest action U;
    - Move it from the *Trial* to the *Alive* set with $V(p) = U(p)$;
    - Update $l(p)$ with the same index as point A_1 in formula (6.6). If $R(A_1) \neq R(B_1)$ and we are in case 1 of section 6.2.4 where both points are used and if this is the first time regions of labels $l(A_1)$ and $l(B_1)$ meet, $S(R_{l(A_1)}, R_{l(B_1)}) = p$ is set as a *saddle point* between $R_{l(A_1)}$ and $R_{l(B_1)}$. If adding a link between these regions does not create a *cycle*, they are set as *linked regions* and $S(R_{l(A_1)}, R_{l(B_1)}) = p$ is selected,

      For each neighbor (i, j) of (i_{min}, j_{min}):
        * If (i, j) is *Far*, add it to the *Trial* set;
        * If (i, j) is *Trial*, update action $U_{i,j}$.
- Obtain all paths between selected *linked regions* by backpropagation each way from their *saddle point* (see Section 6.3.5).

Table 6.2. Algorithm of Section 6.3

point p on the boundary between L_j and L_k, we have $\mathcal{U}_{R_k}(p) = \mathcal{U}_{R_j}(p)$. The *saddle point* $S(R_k, R_j)$ is a point on this boundary with minimal value of $\mathcal{U}_{R_k}(p) = \mathcal{U}_{R_j}(p)$. This gives us a rule to find the *saddle points* during the fast marching algorithm.

Each time two fronts coming from R_k and R_j meet for the first time, we define the meeting point as $S(R_k, R_j)$. This means that we need to know for each point of the image from where it comes. This is easy to keep track of its origin by generating an index map updated at each time a point is set as alive in the algorithm. Each point of region R_k starts with label k. Each time a point is set as alive, it gets the same label as the points it was computed from in formula (6.6). In that formula, the computation of $U_{i,j}$ depends only on at most two of the four pixels involved. These two pixels, said A_1 and B_1, have to be with the same *label*, except if (i, j) is on the boundary between two labels. If A_1 and B_1 are both alive and with different labels k and l, this means that regions R_k and R_l meet there. If this happens for the first time, the current point is set as the *saddle point* $S(R_k, R_l)$ between these regions. A point on the boundary between R_k and R_l is given the label of the neighbor point with smaller action A_1. At the boundary between two labels there can be a slight error on labeling. This error of at most one pixel is not important in our context and could be refined if necessary.

6.3.6   Algorithm

The algorithm for this section is described in Table 6.2 and illustrated in figures 6.3 to 6.5. When there is a large number of R_k's, this does not change much the computation time of the minimal action map, but this makes more complex dealing with the list of linked regions and *saddle points* and testing for *cycles*.

The way we chose to test for cycles is as follows. Assume a saddle point between regions R_i and R_j is found. We then test if there is already a link between these regions through other regions. This means we are looking for a sequence of different regions $R_k, 1 \leq k \leq K$, with $R_1 = R_i$ and $R_K = R_j$, such that for $1 \leq k \leq K - 1$, R_k and R_{k+1} are *linked regions*.

This kind of condition can be easily implemented using a recursive algorithm. When two regions R_i and R_j are willing to be connected - ie that their fronts meet - a table storing the connectivity between each region enables to detect if a link already exists between those regions. Having N different regions, we fill a matrix $M(N, N)$ with zeros, and each time two regions R_i and R_j meet without creating a cycle, we set $M(i, j) = M(j, i) = 1$. Thus, when two regions meet, we apply the algorithm detailed in table 6.3.

Algorithm for Cycle detection when a region R_i meets a region R_j:
$Test(i, j, M, i); with$
$Test(i, j, M, l);$

- if $M(l, j) = 1$, return 1;
- else
  - count=0;
  - for $k \in [1, N]$ with $k \neq i, k \neq j, k \neq l$: count $+= Test(k, j, M, l);$
  - return count;

Table 6.3. Cycle detection

If two regions are already linked, the pixel where their fronts meet is not considered as a valuable candidate for back-propagation. The algorithm stops automatically when all regions are connected.

6.3.7   Application

The method can be applied to connected components from a whole set of edge points or points obtained through a preprocessing. Finding all paths from a given set of points is interesting in the case of a binary potential defined, like in Figure 6.3, for perceptual grouping. It can be used as well when a special preprocessing is possible, either on the image itself to extract characteristic points or on the geometry of the initial set of points to choose more relevant points. We show in Figure 6.6 an example of application for a hip medical image where we are looking for vessels. Potential P is defined using ideas from [8] on vesselness filter (detailed later in section 6.4.2).

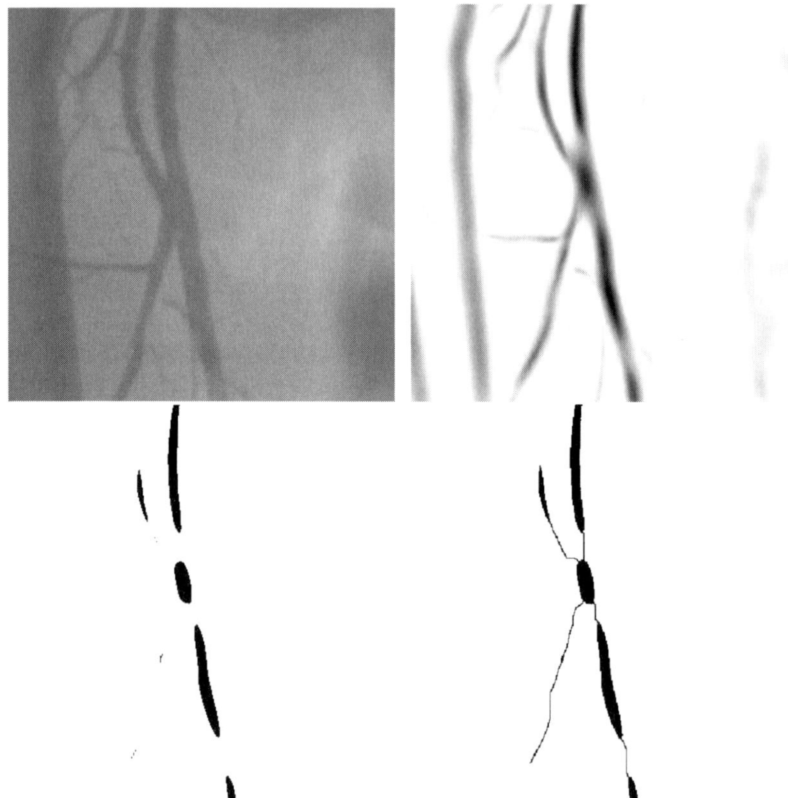

Fig. 6.6. Medical Image. First line: original image and vesselness potential; Second line: from the set of regions obtained from thresholding of potential image, our method finds links between these regions as minimal paths with respect to the potential.

6.4   Finding a Set of Paths in a 3D Image

6.4.1   Extension to 3D

We now extend our approach to finding a set of 3D minimal paths between regions in 3D images. All definitions and algorithms of section 6.3 are not affected by changing the dimension of the image from 2D to 3D. The main changes are that 4-connexity in 2D is now 6-connexity in 3D and that we deal with minimal paths and minimal action in 3D images. We presented briefly in section 6.2.5 the fast marching extension to 3D and for more details on minimal paths in 3D images, we refer to [5] and [6].

6.4.2   Application to Real Datasets: a MR Image of the Aorta

The problem here is to complete a partially detected object. In figure 6.7 is shown a 3D MR dataset of the aorta, which presents a typical pathology: an abdominal aortic aneurysm. The anatomical object is made visible on the image by injecting a contrast product before the image acquisition.

We propose here to give a method for extracting from the grey level image a set of paths that will represent an approximate skeleton of the tree structure. This is based on extracting first a set of unstructured voxels or regions that belong to the object.

For this, we propose to extract valuable information from this dataset, computing a multiscale vessel enhancement measure, based on the work of [8] on ridge filters. Having extracted the three eigenvalues of the Hessian matrix computed at scale σ, ordered $|\lambda_1| \le |\lambda_2| \le |\lambda_3|$, we define a vesselness function

$$\nu(s) = \begin{cases} 0, \text{ if } \lambda_2 \ge 0 \text{ or } \lambda_3 \ge 0 \\ (1 - \exp \frac{-R_A{}^2}{2\alpha^2}) \exp \frac{-R_B{}^2}{2\beta^2} (1 - \exp \frac{-S^2}{2c^2}) \text{ else} \end{cases}$$

where $R_A = \frac{|\lambda_2|}{|\lambda_3|}$, $R_B = \frac{|\lambda_1|}{\sqrt{|\lambda_2 \lambda_3|}}$, and $S = \sqrt{\lambda_1{}^2 + \lambda_2{}^2 + \lambda_3{}^2}$. See [8] for a detailed explanation of the settings of each parameter in this measure.

In figure 6.8 you can observe the response of the filter, based on the Hessian information, at three different scales: $\sigma = 1, 5, 10$. Visualization is made with Maximum Intensity Projection (MIP). Using this information computed at several scales, we can take as potential the maximum of the response of the filter across all scales which is shown also in figure 6.8-bottom-right. And we can easily give a very constrained threshold of this image, that will lead to sets of unstructured voxels that surely belong to the anatomical object of interest, as shown in figure 6.9-left.

Based on this set of regions, we apply our algorithm of section 6.3, using the 3D version of the Fast Marching algorithm presented briefly in section 6.2.5 and which is detailed in [6]. We find the set of paths that connect altogether all the seed regions in our image, leading to the representation shown in figure 6.9-right.

6.5   Conclusion

We presented a new method that finds a set of contour curves in an image. It was applied to perceptual grouping to get complete curves from a set of edge regions with gaps. The technique is based on finding minimal paths between two end points [4]. However, in our approach, we do not need to give the start and end points as initialization. Given a unstructured set of regions, we found the pairs of regions that had to be linked by minimal paths. Once *saddle points* between pairs of regions are found, paths are drawn on the image from the selected *saddle points* to both points of each pair. This gives the minimal paths between selected pairs of regions. The whole set of paths completes the initial set of contours and allows to close these contours. We applied this method in order to reconstruct vascular structures, and we showed examples for 2D vascular image and 3D medical dataset of the aorta.

References

1. V. Caselles, R. Kimmel, and G. Sapiro. Geodesic active contours. *IJCV*, 22(1):61–79, 1997.
2. Laurent D. Cohen. On active contour models and balloons. *CVGIP:IU*, 53(2):211–218, March 1991.
3. Laurent D. Cohen. Multiple Contour Finding and Perceptual Grouping using Minimal Paths. Journal of Mathematical Imaging and Vision, 14(3), 2001, to appear.
4. Laurent D. Cohen and R. Kimmel. Global minimum for active contour models: A minimal path approach. *IJCV*, 24(1):57–78, August 1997.
5. T. Deschamps and L. D. Cohen. Minimal paths in 3D images and application to virtual endoscopy. In *Proc. ECCV'00*, Dublin, Ireland, July 2000.
6. T. Deschamps and L. D. Cohen. Fast extraction of minimal paths in 3D images and applications to virtual endoscopy. Medical Image Analysis, 2001, to appear.
7. E. W. Dijkstra. A note on two problems in connection with graphs. *Numerische Math.*, 1:269–271, 1959.
8. A. Frangi and W. Niessen, Multiscale Vessel Enhancement Filtering. MICCAI'98, Cambridge.
9. G. Guy and G. Medioni. Inferring global perceptual contours from local features. *IJCV*, 20(1/2) Oct. 1996.
10. M. Kass, A. Witkin and D. Terzopoulos. Snakes: Active contour models. *IJCV*, 1(4):321–331, Jan. 1988.
11. R. Kimmel, A. Amir, and A. Bruckstein. Finding shortest paths on surfaces using level sets propagation. *IEEE* PAMI-17(6):635–640, June 1995.
12. R. Kimmel, N. Kiryati, and A. M. Bruckstein. Distance maps and weighted distance transforms. *JMIV*, 6:223–233, May 1996.
13. R. Malladi, J. A. Sethian, and B. C. Vemuri. Shape modeling with front propagation: A level set approach. *IEEE PAMI*, 17(2):158–175, february 1995.
14. J. A. Sethian. *Level Set Methods: Evolving Interfaces in Geometry, Fluid Mechanics, Computer Vision and Materials Sciences.* Cambridge Univ. Press, 1996.
15. A. Shaashua and S. Ullman. Structural saliency: The detection of globally salient structures using a locally connected network. In *Proc. ICCV'88*, Dec. 1988.
16. L. R. Williams and D. W. Jacobs. stochastic completion fields: a neural model of illusory contour shape and salience. In *Proc. ICCV'95*, June 1995.

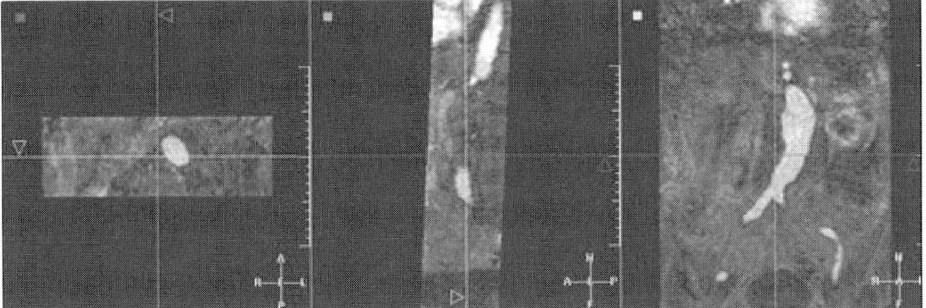

Fig. 6.7. Three orthogonal slices of the aorta MR dataset

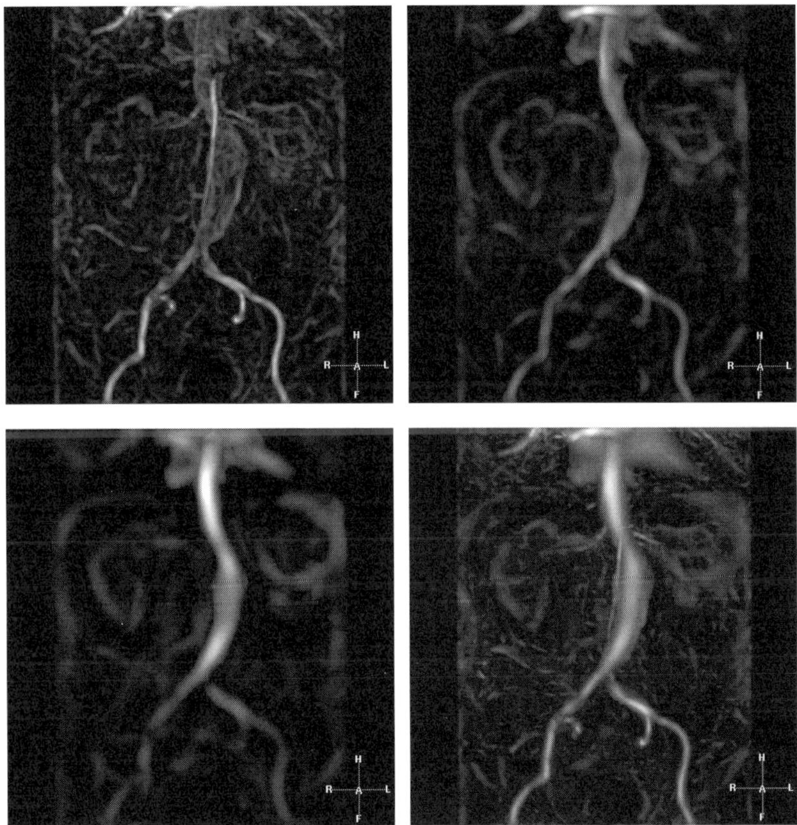

Fig. 6.8. From left to right and bottom to down: Ridge detection at three different scales ($\sigma = 1, 5, 10$), and resulting 3D potential (MIP visualization of the 3D images)

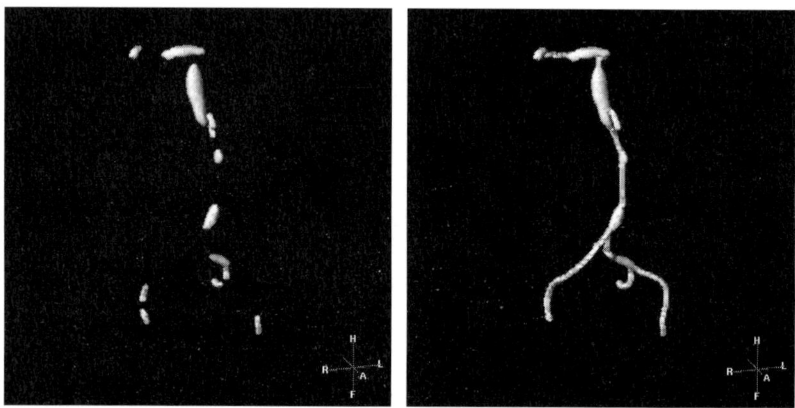

Fig. 6.9. Perceptual Grouping in the aorta of figure 6.7: from left to right, a rough detection of the aorta; the Reconstructed aorta.

7 Nonlinear Multiscale Analysis Models for Filtering of 3D + Time Biomedical Images

A. Sarti[1], K. Mikula[2], F. Sgallari[3], and C. Lamberti[1]

[1] DEIS, University of Bologna, Italy
[2] Department of Mathematics, Slovak University of Technology, Radlinskeho 11, 813 68 Bratislava, Slovakia
[3] Department of Mathematics, University of Bologna, Italy

Abstract. We review nonlinear partial differential equations (PDEs) in the processing of 2D and 3D images. At the same time we present recent models introduced for processing of space-time image sequences and apply them to 3D echocardiography. The nonlinear (degenerate) diffusion equations filter the sequence with a keeping of space-time coherent structures. They have been developed using ideas of regularized Perona-Malik anisotropic diffusion and geometrical diffusion of mean curvature flow type, combined with Galilean invariant movie multiscale analysis of Alvarez, Guichard, Lions and Morel. A discretization of space-time filtering equations is discussed. Computational results in processing of 3D echocardiographic sequences obtained by rotational acquisition technique and by Real-Time 3D Echo Volumetrics aquisition technique are presented.

7.1 Introduction

The aim of this contribution is to present mathematical models, numerical methods and computational results in processing of three-dimensional (3D) image sequences. We apply the proposed models and methods to 3D echocardiography. The models which we use for space-time filtering are based on partial differential equations (PDEs) approach, namely PDEs of degenerate diffusion type are applied to initially given image sequence. Since the images are given on discrete grids, the nonlinear PDEs are discretized by semi-implicit finite volume method in order to get fast and stable solution.

Two-dimensional (2D) echocardiography is an imaging modality frequently used in cardiology due to its simplicity, lack of ionizing radiation and a relative low cost. However, 2D echocardiography allows visualization of only tomographic planar sections of the heart; thus to obtain a complete evaluation of the heart anatomy and function, the physician must reassemble mentally a 3D model from multiple two-dimensional images. Moreover, 2D echocardiography relies on geometrical assumptions for the determination of heart chamber volumes and thus presents a considerable measurement error. 3D echocardiography may avoid the need for geometrical assumptions, thereby allowing accurate evaluation of chambers size and shape, even in the case of cavities with irregular or distorted geometry. The correct visualization and interpretation of 3D echo images is often affected by the high amount of noise intrinsically linked to the acquisition method. It is absolutely necessary to submit the data to pre-processing in order to improve their legibility from a clinical point of view. The pre-processing algorithm should be able to distinguish the noise from the contours of the different cardiac structures by using both spatial and temporal coherence.

In this paper we use two types of 3D echocardiographic data sets to which our algorithms are applied and tested. The first sequence has been obtained by means of a rotational acquisition technique using the TomTec Imaging System. With this technique the transducer undergoes a rotation around its main axis in a propeller configuration. A series of tomographies corresponding to the sections of a cone of biological tissue has been acquired. The acquisition consists of 14 image-cubes that represent a whole cardiac cycle of a real patient. A volume of interest of 150 x 150 x 100 voxels will be processed. The interval of time between one cube and the next one is 40 ms. Figures 7.1-7.3, 7.6-7.7 are related to results on this data set. The quality of this 3D raw dataset is quite good. Nevertheless a remarkable amount of noise is present in the sequence and thus it is reasonable testing example for the proposed methods. The second type of processed data is given by real 3D ultrasound echo-images. Real-Time 3D Echo (RT3DE Volumetrics) acqusition technique is characterized by a 43 x 43 piezoelectric elements transducer with 2.5 - 3.5 MHz frequency, 60 x 60 degree angular opening and 256 transmission lines. There are 64×64 pixels in each of 512 C-scan planes and 2097152 voxels in every 3D frame. The main difference between RT3DE and 2D rotational acquisition is that RT3DE can provide images of left ventricle without ECG/respiratory gating, there is less acquisition time and no processing time. RT3DE can be used also in arrhytmia cases and no special training is required. However there is less resolution because of broadened transmit pattern.

From mathematical point of view, the input image sequence, representing an acquizition of moving objects, can be modelled by a real function $u^0(x, \theta)$, $u^0 : \Omega \times [0, T] \to I\!\!R$, where $\Omega \subset I\!\!R^N$ represents a spatial domain, $x = (x_1, \ldots, x_N)$ represents a spatial point and θ a point in the time interval $[0, T]$ in which acquizition is realized. In practice, Ω is rectangular domain, $N = 2$ or 3 and, in special applications, the time sequence can be periodically prolonged from $[0, T]$ to $I\!\!R$. The typical example which can be represented by such u^0 is an ultrasound acquizition of beating heart in 3D echocardiography (see numerical examples in next sections). The application of PDE to initially given (noisy) image sequence can be understood as its embedding to the so-called *nonlinear scale space*. The axioms and fundamental properties of such embedding has been given and studied in [1] and the notion of *image multiscale analysis* has been introduced. The image multiscale analysis associates with u^0 a family $u(t, x, \theta)$ of smoothed - simplified images (in our case a family of smoothed sequences) depending on an abstract parameter t, the *scale*. As it has been proved in [1], if such family fulfills basic assumptions - pyramidal structure, regularity and local comparison principle - then $u(t, x, \theta)$, $u : [0, T_s] \times \Omega \times [0, T] \rightarrow I\!R$ can be represented as unique viscosity solution of a second order (degenerate) parabolic partial differential equation

$$\frac{\partial u}{\partial t} = F(t, u, Du, D^2 u) \tag{7.1}$$

with the initial condition given by $u(0, x, \theta) = u^0(x, \theta)$. The equations of (degenerate) parabolic type has a smoothing property, so they are natural tool for filtering (image simplification) by removing spurious structures, e.g. a noise. However, the simplification should be "image oriented", e.g. it should respect edges and do not blur them. Or, it should recognize motion of a structure in image sequence and consequently the smoothing (diffusion) should respect the motion coherence in subsequent frames. Such, or even more sofisticated requirements related to geometrical characteristics of image, bring strong nonlinearity into the parabolic PDEs (diffusion can depend on $|\nabla u|$ - edge indicator) or even degeneracy (diffusion can be stopped in points which are "un-noisy" by motion field information).

In Section 2, the models for processing of 2D and 3D images based on anisotropic Perona-Malik type diffusion and geometrical diffusion of mean curvature flow type are given. We discuss their main features related to image selective smoothing and give references to works describing efficient computational methods. In Section 3, we present models for space-time filtering which combines spatial diffusion equations from Section 2 with motion coherence of moving objects in time. In Section 4 we discuss numerical methods for solving our space-time filtering equations. In Section 5 we present computational results obtained by such schemes in filtering of artificial as well as echocardiographic image sequences.

7.2   Nonlinear Diffusion Equations for Processing of 2D and 3D Still Images

In this section we give an overview of nonlinear diffusion equations used for processing frames of the sequence independently on each other. In the next chapter such spatial smoothing processes will be combined with motion coherence in entire image sequence. Let $v^0(x) = u(0, x, \theta^*)$ be a frame of initially given image sequence at some time moment $\theta^* \in [0, T]$.

7.2.1   Anisotropic diffusion of Perona-Malik type

From the end of eighties, the nonlinear diffusion equations have been used for processing of 2D and 3D images. After pioneering work of Perona and Malik ([14]) who made generalization of linear heat equation (equivalent to Gaussian smoothing) to nonlinear diffusion preserving edge positions, the large interest in application and analysis of such equations started. At present, the following nonlinear partial differential equation ([4]) is widely used

$$v_t - \nabla.(g(|\nabla G_\sigma * v|)\nabla v) = 0, \tag{7.2}$$

where $v(t,x)$ is unknown function defined in $Q_{T_s} \equiv [0,T_s] \times \Omega$. We assume that $\Omega \subset I\!\!R^N$ is a bounded rectangular domain, $[0,T_s]$ is scaling interval and $g : I\!\!R_0^+ \to I\!\!R^+$ is a nonincreasing smooth function, $g(0) = 1$, $g(s) \to 0$ for $s \to \infty$. In equation (7.2), $G_\sigma \in C^\infty(I\!\!R^N)$ is a smoothing kernel (e.g. Gauss function) with unit mass and tending to Dirac function as $\sigma \to 0$. The convolution in (7.2) is understood in the usual sense

$$\nabla G_\sigma * v = \int_{I\!\!R^N} \nabla G_\sigma(x - \xi)\tilde{v}(\xi)d\xi, \tag{7.3}$$

where $\tilde{v}$ is an extension of v to $I\!\!R^N$ given by a periodic reflection through the boundary of Ω. The equation (7.2) is accompanied with zero Neumann boundary conditions and initial condition

$$\frac{\partial v}{\partial \nu} = 0 \quad \text{on } [0,T_s] \times \partial\Omega, \tag{7.4}$$

$$v(0,x) = v^0(x) \quad \text{in } \Omega, \quad v^0 \in L_\infty(\Omega), \tag{7.5}$$

where ν is unit normal vector to the boundary of Ω. The equation (7.2) represents a modification of the well-known Perona-Malik equation ([14])

$$v_t - \nabla.(g(|\nabla v|)\nabla v) = 0, \tag{7.6}$$

called also *anisotropic diffusion* in computer vision community. It was introduced in context of nonlinear image filtration, edge detection, image enhancement, restoration and segmentation. The equation selectively diffuses image in the regions where the signal has small variance in intensity in contrast with those regions where the signal changes its tendency. Such diffusion process is governed by the shape of diffusion coefficient given by the function g and by its dependence on ∇v which is understood as an edge indicator ([14]). Since $g \to 0$ for large gradients the diffusion is slowed down on edges. As one can see, in the original Perona-Malik formulation (7.6), ∇v stands in place of the convolution term $\nabla G_\sigma * v$ of equation (7.2). However, in such original form the Perona-Malik equation can behave locally like backward heat equation which is an ill-posed problem solvability of which is a difficult problem ([10]). Catté, Lions, Morel and Coll in [4] introduced the convolution with Gaussian kernel G_σ into the decision process for the value of the diffusion coefficient. Such slight modification allowed to prove existence and uniqueness of the weak solution for the modified equation and to keep practical advantages of original formulation.

Since an image is given on a discrete grid we discretize PDE to get a numerical scheme implemented on computer. One can use wide range of methods devoted to numerical solution of PDEs. The semi-implicit schemes ([4], [9], [3], [12], [21]), where nonlinear terms of equation are treated from the previous discrete scale step and linear terms are considered on the current scale level, have favourable stability and efficiency properties and they converge to the weak solution of the parabolic problem (7.2)-(7.5) ([9], [12]). For space discretization either finite element method ([9], [3]), finite volume method ([12]) or finite difference method ([4], [21]) can be used. For discretization details by variational methods we refer to [8]. Here we present application of semi-implicit finite element method to 3D echocardiographic image of one moment of cardiac cycle with left ventricle in open phase (using TomTec data set). In Figure 7.1, one can see visualization of the isosurface representing boundary between blood and muscle, forming an edge in 3D image intensity, in subsequent discrete scale steps of semi-implicit method. The experiment is taken from [3]. The image intensity is smoothed out of edge and edge itself is well kept. However, since final state of diffusion process given by (7.2) is *constant* given by mean value of initial image, in general situation there is no guarrantee of reasonable *stopping time* T_s which one has to choose in order to stop filtering. This disadvantage can be weaken using motion field information from dynamic sequence as we will explain in Section 7.3.

7.2.2   Geometrical diffusion of mean curvature flow type

In [13], [7] we applied another type of diffusion to 3D echocardiographic frames. We call it geometrical diffusion since it is related to geometrical (or intrinsic) diffusion equations on manifolds. In rather general situations, the blood - cardiac muscle interface corresponds to an isosurface (isoline in 2D) of the greylevel image intensity function and hence it forms recognizable silhouette in the image. This phenomcnon is transparently visible in Figure 7.2. To remove an un-smoothness of the silhouette (in the original image or in the prefiltered by anisotropic diffusion image) caused by errors in acquisition, it seems reasonable to move such iso-surface (iso-curve) in direction of its normal vector field with the velocity proportional to the mean curvature. The motions of convex and concave pieces are opposite due to the curvature sign, and the large fingers shrink much more faster than smoother parts due to the curvature dependence of the flow. Thus, locally in scale, we can obtain desirable smoothing of the silhouette. This idea was used also in [2], where equation

$$v_t - g(|\nabla G_\sigma * v|)|\nabla v|\nabla.(\frac{\nabla v}{|\nabla v|}) = 0, \tag{7.7}$$

has been suggested for computational image and shape analysis. Provided $g \equiv 1$, (7.7) is called the level set equation suggested by Osher and Sethian for computing an evolving front in interfacial dynamics. From practical point

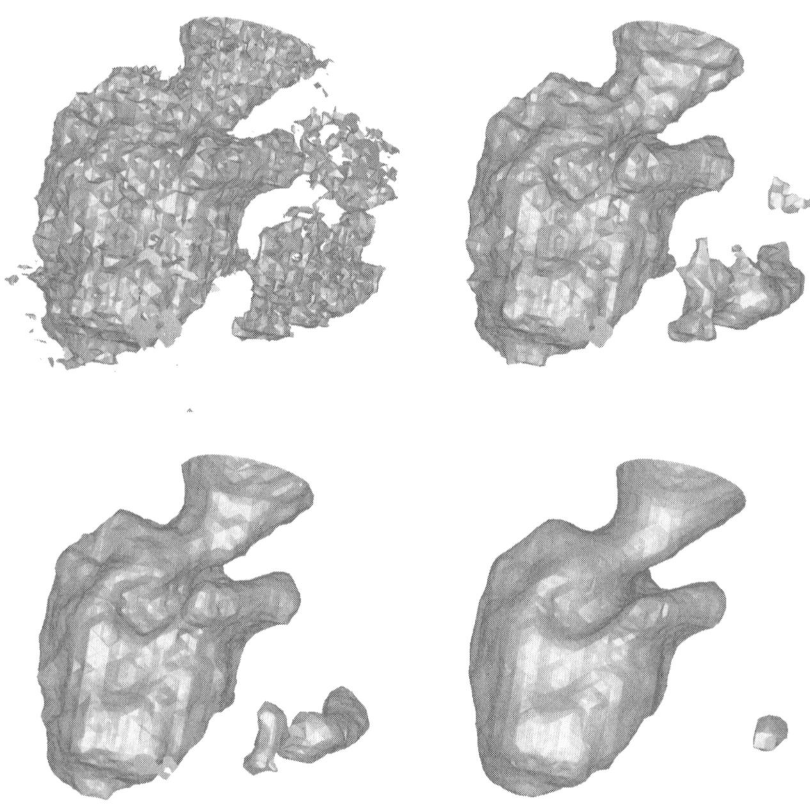

Fig. 7.1. Smoothing of the human left ventricle by anisotropic diffusion. We visualize correponding level surfaces in 0th, 2nd, 4th and 8th discrete steps of semi-implicit finite element algorithm ([3])

of view, applying just the level set equation to initial image yields the intrinsic silhouettes smoothing ([13], [7]). On the other hand, equation (7.7) can be used successively for image selective smoothing with preserving edge positions in a similar way like equation (7.2). The Perona-Malik function $g(s)$ depending on $|\nabla G_\sigma * v|$ is used to strongly slowing down the motion of the silhouettes which are at the same time un-spurious edges. The regions between them are smoothed by the mean curvature flow. In case of geometrical diffusion we again consider zero Neumann boundary conditions on $\partial\Omega$ and initial condition given by processed image v^0. A 2D and 3D filtering algorithm has been also proposed in [18] where the level set equation has been rewritten with respect to a Riemannian metric induced by the image.

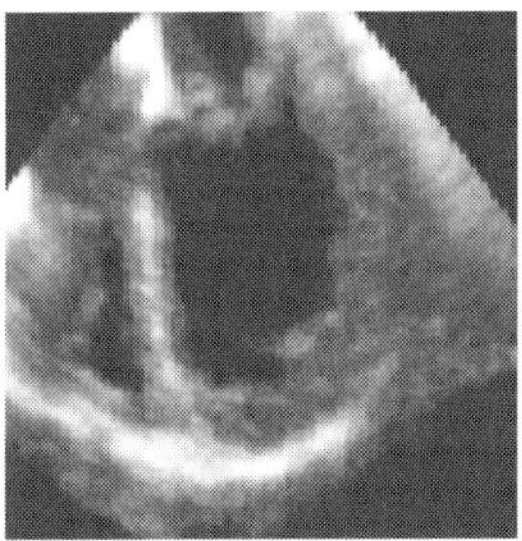 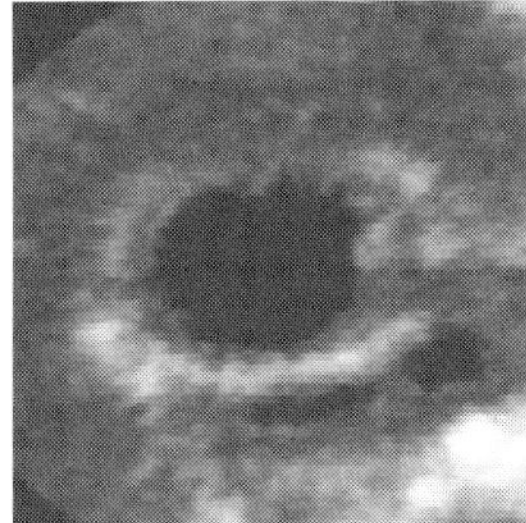 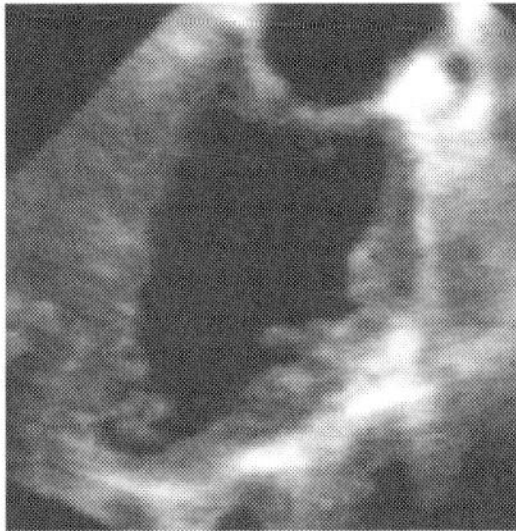

Fig. 7.2. 2D cuts of 3D echocardiographic cube with image of the human left ventricle

The level-set-like equations are degenerate parabolic and hence rather complicated from the numerical point of view. Its solution can be tracked e.g. by the well-known level set method based on a solution of first order Hamilton-Jacobi equation ([20]). However in curvature driven motion one can use also another approach leading to usage of standard numerical methods for solving parabolic PDEs, namely finite clement or finite volume methods for discretization in space and semi-implicit method in scale ([13], [7], [8]). Such approach is L_∞-stable and leads to solving of linear systems in every discrete scale level. Hence one can use state-of-the-art methods of numerical linear algebra and preconditioners.

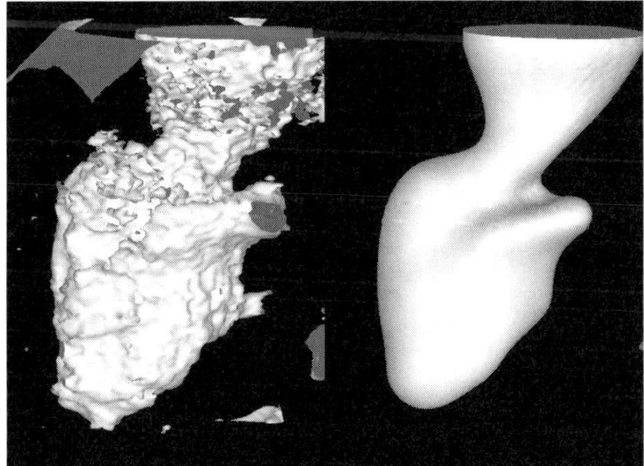

Fig. 7.3. Ventricular shape extraction using geometrical diffusion.

We present application of geometrical diffusion to medical image processing obtaining a smooth shape of the left heart ventricle. In Figure 7.3 we visualize the level surfaces which represent the boundary of the volume containing the blood in a discrete moment of cardiac cycle from the TomTec

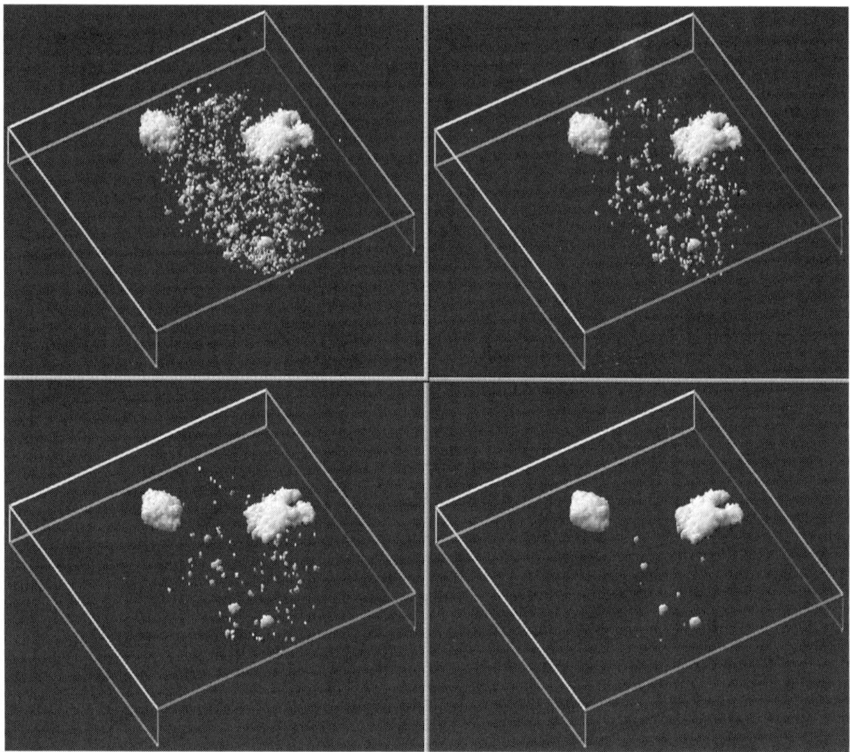

Fig. 7.4. Extraction of two chromozomes in human cell using geometrical diffusion.

testing data set (processing of 5th frame of the sequence is presented). On the left side, the unfiltered isosurface is plotted. In right side, we present computational result after 21 discrete scale steps on Cray C92. For longer time-scale the diffusion tends to shrink the structure. This shortcomming of the method will be improved by considering space-time coherence of the entire sequence given in the next section. We present also Figure 7.4 where two chromozomes are extracted from initial noisy 3D-image of human cell by image selective smoothing (7.7) with $g(s) = 1/(1 + s^2)$.

In the end of this section, let us mention a general usefull view to gradient dependent nonlinear (geometrical) diffusion equations. The nonlinear diffusion term $\nabla.(g(|\nabla u|)\nabla u)$ can be rewritten in 2D as

$$\nabla.(g(|\nabla u|)\nabla u) = g(|\nabla u|)u_{\xi\xi} + H'(|\nabla u|)u_{\eta\eta} \qquad (7.8)$$

where $H(s) = sg(s)$ and ξ, η are tangential and orthogonal vectors to the level line, respectively. From this form one can simply see how diffusion works along and across the image silhouettes with different choices of g. There is always positive, but possibly strongly slowed-down diffusion along level lines. Across level line there can be forward diffusion (when $H'(s)$ is positive), zero diffusion (e.g. in Rudin-Osher-Fatemi model [15] dealing with total variation denoising and also in the mean curvature flow equation in the level set formulation) or backward diffusion (in the original Perona-Malik model [14], [10]).

7.3   Space-Time Filtering Nonlinear Diffusion Equations

A 3D space-time image sequence (e.g. in 3D echocardiography) $u^0(x,\theta)$ is a 4D image and we can apply general multiscale analysis model (7.1) to it. The question is how to choose right hand side of (7.1) with the aim to extract relevant information from the sequence, filter out the noise and enhance moving structures. To that goal we would like to use an additional information (in comparison with the still image processing) given by motion coherence in the image sequence. We will assume that certain objects acquired in different time, and thus being in different frames of the sequence, are formed by points that preserve their intensity along the motion trajectory. Such objects are called Lambertian structures. Moreover we assume that motion is Galilean locally in time, i.e. the motion trajectories are smooth. Designing the model equations we will consider the following quantity proposed by Guichard ([1],[6])

$$clt(u) = \min_{w_1,w_2} (|<\nabla u, w_1 - w_2>|+ \tag{7.9}$$

$$|u(t, x - w_1, \theta - \Delta\theta) - u(t, x, \theta)| + |u(t, x + w_2, \theta + \Delta\theta) - u(t, x, \theta)|)$$

where w_1, w_2 are arbitrary vectors in $I\!\!R^N$ and $\Delta\theta$ is the time increment. The scalar function $clt(u)$ (the name clt indicates the relation to the curvature of Lambertian trajectory) will introduce a measure of coherence in time for the moving structures. It consists of the sum of three positive parts and we want to find the minimum in all possible directions w_1, w_2. The last two terms in the sum on the right hand side of (7.9) are related to the differences in the intensities of end-points of candidate Lambertian velocity vectors w_1, w_2. To find the directions of such vectors we look at the points which have the closest intensity value to the intensity $u(t, x, \theta)$ in the previous frame (term $|u(t, x - w_1, \theta - \Delta\theta) - u(t, x, \theta)|$) and in the next frame (term $|u(t, x + w_2, \theta + \Delta\theta) - u(t, x, \theta)|$). Note that, if we find corresponding Lambertian points both terms vanish. The first term in the sum, namely $|<\nabla u, w_1 - w_2>|$, corresponds to the so called *apparent acceleration*, i.e. to the difference between candidate Lambertian velocity vectors w_1 and w_2 in the direction of ∇u. For details and some more background from the optic flow we refer to [1], [6]. One can say that quantity $clt(u)$ is related to the curvature of the space-time level curve passing through the space-time point (x, θ) in the scale t. The value of $clt(u)$ vanishes for the Lambertian points that are in Galilean motion. It is consistent with our purposes to not alter such trajectories. On the other hand for the noisy points there is no motion coherence and thus $clt(u)$ will be large there.

Concerning the space coherence, we assume that distinguished structures are located in the regions with a certain mean value of the image intensity function and that object boundary forms an edge in the image. In order to construct spatial diffusion process we will require specific behavior on the edges, e.g. it is desirable not to blur them, to keep their position as fixed as possible. Another reasonable choice can be related to a smoothing of the edges by intrinsic diffusion (for that goal, flow by mean curvature can be used). There exist diffusion processes designed to respect such features (see Section 2); we can choose e.g Perona-Malik like anisotropic diffusion, mean curvature flow of curves and surfaces in the level set fomulation, models based on minimization of image total variation etc.

To combine time coherence of moving objects with their spatial localization we consider the following equation

$$\frac{\partial u}{\partial t} = clt(u) \ sd(u) \tag{7.10}$$

where spatial diffusion is given either by the Perona–Malik term, i.e.

$$sd(u) = \nabla.(g(|\nabla u|)\nabla u) \tag{7.11}$$

or by level set like term, i.e.

$$sd(u) = |\nabla u|\nabla.\left(\frac{\nabla u}{|\nabla u|}\right). \tag{7.12}$$

To prevent possible degeneracies we will regularize the equations. As explained in Section 2, the Perona–Malik diffusion equation is well-posed only under assumption $g(s) + g'(s)s \geq 0$. However, it is usual to use function g as

$$g(s) = \frac{1}{1 + Ks^2} \tag{7.13}$$

with some constant K. To preveal ill-posedness of equation in such case we use spatial regularization by smoothing kernel due to [4]. In case of Perona–Malik spatial smoothing we have proposed the following equation for the processing of image sequences ([17])

$$\frac{\partial u}{\partial t} = clt(u)\nabla.(g(|\nabla G_\sigma * u|)\nabla u). \tag{7.14}$$

The practical choice of the kernel is N-dimensional Gauss function

$$G_\sigma(x) = \frac{1}{(2\sqrt{\pi\sigma})^N}e^{-\frac{|x|^2}{4\sigma}}. \tag{7.15}$$

In the second case (7.12), i.e. when we are interested in the smoothing of moving object silhouette by intrinsic diffusion we use regularization in the sense of Evans and Spruck and thus consider the equation

$$\frac{\partial u}{\partial t} = clt(u)\sqrt{\varepsilon^2 + |\nabla u|^2}\nabla.\left(\frac{\nabla u}{\sqrt{\varepsilon^2 + |\nabla u|^2}}\right) \qquad (7.16)$$

where ε is a small regularization parameter. In both cases, (7.14) and (7.16), we consider zero Neumann boundary conditions in the spatial part of boundary and e.g. periodic boundary conditions in time boundary of the sequence.

In the models (7.14) and (7.16), the change of image intensity in scale, i.e. $\frac{\partial u}{\partial t}$, is given by the right hand side of (7.14) or (7.16). There the spatial diffusion term is multiplied by $clt(u)$. Thus, the diffusion process degenerates (is stopped) in the Lambertian points that are in Galilean motion. It is an important difference from standard selective smoothing processes for still images. We can conclude that, the equations (7.14), (7.16) preserve moving in time structures as well as keep (or slightly smooth) their spatial edges.

7.4   Numerical Algorithm

In this section we describe a method for numerical solution of image sequence multiscale analysis equations (7.14) and (7.16). Let our space-time sequence consists of $m + 1$ frames. Let $\vartheta = \Delta\theta = \frac{T}{m}$ be a discrete time step of the sequence (without lost of generality, let us have $\vartheta = 1$). Let us denote a discrete scale step by τ. Then by u_j^i we denote the j-th frame of the sequence in i-th discrete scale step, i.e.

$$u_j^i(x_1, x_2, x_3) = u(i\tau, x_1, x_2, x_3, j\vartheta). \qquad (7.17)$$

The basic idea of our numerical method is to handle terms in (7.14) or (7.16) in such a way to obtain a linear boundary value problem for u_j^i. The reason is that such equations can be solved by robust and efficient spatial discretization techniques based on finite volume (FVM), finite difference (FDM) or finite element methods (FEM). To that goal, the nonlinearities of equation (7.14) are treated using the previous scale step, while the linear terms are handled implicitly. Such approach is called semi-implicit approximation in scale. Then we provide space-time discretization and, finally, our numerical method leads to solving of linear algebraic systems in order to update each frame of the sequence in a new scale.

Let us discuss the discretization of the terms in (7.14). From definition (7.9), we can obtain a time-discrete version of $clt(u)$ considering current, previous and next time frame of the sequence. We define

$$clt(u_j^i) = \min_{w_1, w_2}(| < \nabla u_j^i, w_1 - w_2 > | + \qquad (7.18)$$

$$|u_{j-1}^i(x - w_1) - u_j^i(x)| + |u_{j+1}^i(x + w_2) - u_j^i(x)|).$$

and we can write **semi-implicit scheme** for solving (7.14):

Let τ and σ be given outer and inner discrete scale steps. For $i = 1, 2, ...$ and for each frame $j = 0, ..., m$ we look for u_j^i satisfying

$$\frac{u_j^i - u_j^{i-1}}{\tau} = clt(u_j^{i-1})\nabla.(g(|\nabla G_\sigma * u_j^{i-1}|)\nabla u_j^i) \tag{7.19}$$

where e.g. the periodicity in time of the sequence is used for $j = 0$ and $j = m$ and the zero Neumann boundary conditions are considered for spatial boundary Ω. Let us mention that, we can use also other conditions for updating the first and last frame in the sequence, e.g. reflexive if we have given only one half of periodic cycle, or first and last frame can serve as Dirichlet data for computing u_j^i, $j = 1, j = m - 1$. Provided (7.15), we can realize the convolution, involved in computing of diffusion coefficient $g(|\nabla G_\sigma * u_j^{i-1}|)$, by solving numerically the linear heat equation

$$\frac{\partial w}{\partial t} = \nabla.(\nabla w) \tag{7.20}$$

in time interval $[0, \sigma]$ with the initial condition $w(x, 0) = u_j^{i-1}(x)$. Then we put $u_j^\sigma := w(x, \sigma)$. Numerically, we solve the equation (7.20) implicitely in t with just one discrete inner scale step with the length σ. So, (7.19) can be rewritten into the couple

$$\frac{u_j^i - u_j^{i-1}}{\tau} = clt(u_j^{i-1})\nabla.(g(|\nabla u_j^\sigma|)\nabla u_j^i) \tag{7.21}$$

where u_j^σ is the solution of

$$\frac{u_j^\sigma - u_j^{i-1}}{\sigma} = \nabla.(\nabla u_j^\sigma) \tag{7.22}$$

$$j = 0, ..., m, \quad i = 1, 2, ...$$

In discrete settings, $\min\limits_{w_1, w_2}$ in (7.18) is evaluated only for vectors connecting pixel/voxel centers P representing nodes of the computational grid (see also [6]). In practice, we look only to a certain (not too large) rectangular neighbourhood centered in P. For space discretization of (7.21) as well as (7.22) we use the so called finite (or control) volume method. Let the discrete image intensity values be given in central points P of finite volumes corresponding to voxels in 3D. Let the distance between two of such points be h (we consider uniform 3D grid) Let us denote the grid neighbours of P by W (west), E (east), S (south), N (north), B (bottom), U (up) and the points crossing the finite volume in the direction of neighbours by w, e, s, n, b, u. The finite volume arround P then can be written as $\mathcal{V} = [w, e] \times [s, n] \times [b, u] \subset I\!\!R^3$. Integrating the equation (7.21) in finite volume $\mathcal{V}$, assuming constant profile of $clt(u_j^{i-1})$ in $\mathcal{V}$, constant diffusion fluxes through boundaries of $\mathcal{V}$, and approximating partial derivatives on the boundaries of finite volume by central differences we obtain following difference equation holding in every P

$$-a_W u_j^i(W) - a_S u_j^i(S) - a_B u_j^i(B) + a_P u_j^i(P) - \qquad (7.23)$$
$$-a_E u_j^i(E) - a_N u_j^i(N) - a_U u_j^i(U) = b_P$$

where

$$a_W = \frac{\tau}{h^2} clt(u_j^{i-1})(P) g(|\nabla u_j^\sigma|)(w), a_E = \frac{\tau}{h^2} clt(u_j^{i-1})(P) g(|\nabla u_j^\sigma|)(e),$$
$$a_S = \frac{\tau}{h^2} clt(u_j^{i-1})(P) g(|\nabla u_j^\sigma|)(s), a_N = \frac{\tau}{h^2} clt(u_j^{i-1})(P) g(|\nabla u_j^\sigma|)(n),$$
$$a_B = \frac{\tau}{h^2} clt(u_j^{i-1})(P) g(|\nabla u_j^\sigma|)(b), a_U = \frac{\tau}{h^2} clt(u_j^{i-1})(P) g(|\nabla u_j^\sigma|)(u),$$
$$a_P = a_W + a_E + a_S + a_N + a_B + a_U + 1, b_P = u_j^{i-1}(P). \qquad (7.24)$$

Applying the zero Neumann boundary conditions to boundary volumes we can represent the equations (7.23) in matrix form

$$\mathbf{A}\bar{u}_j^i = \bar{b} \qquad (7.25)$$

where $\bar{u}_j^i$ represents the vector of unknown discrete values of u_j^i in the grid nodes. The coefficients of the matrix $\mathbf{A}$ depend on u_j^σ and u_j^{i-1} and thus they are recomputed in each discrete frame and scale step. Because of the dependence on u_j^σ, we have to solve inner equation (7.22). The finite volume method for (7.22) leads to linear system with the symmetric matrix which is same in each frame and scale step. Hence we simply obtain the vector $\bar{u}_j^\sigma$ i.e. values of u_j^σ in grid points. Using those values, we compute the approximate value of $g(|\nabla u_j^\sigma|)$ for each crossing finite volume boundary point $w, e, \ldots$ Finally we arrange the matrix $\mathbf{A}$. The system (7.25) is then solved by efficient linear algebraic solver. Using the similar ideas we obtain the discrete version of the equation (7.16), the linear system of type (7.25) with coefficients

$$a_W = \frac{\tau}{h^2} clt(u_j^{i-1})(P) \sqrt{\varepsilon^2 + |\nabla u_j^{i-1}|^2}(P) / \sqrt{\varepsilon^2 + |\nabla u_j^{i-1}|^2}(w),$$
$$a_E = \frac{\tau}{h^2} clt(u_j^{i-1})(P) \sqrt{\varepsilon^2 + |\nabla u_j^{i-1}|^2}(P) / \sqrt{\varepsilon^2 + |\nabla u_j^{i-1}|^2}(e),$$
$$a_S = \frac{\tau}{h^2} clt(u_j^{i-1})(P) \sqrt{\varepsilon^2 + |\nabla u_j^{i-1}|^2}(P) / \sqrt{\varepsilon^2 + |\nabla u_j^{i-1}|^2}(s),$$
$$a_N = \frac{\tau}{h^2} clt(u_j^{i-1})(P) \sqrt{\varepsilon^2 + |\nabla u_j^{i-1}|^2}(P) / \sqrt{\varepsilon^2 + |\nabla u_j^{i-1}|^2}(n), \quad (7.26)$$
$$a_B = \frac{\tau}{h^2} clt(u_j^{i-1})(P) \sqrt{\varepsilon^2 + |\nabla u_j^{i-1}|^2}(P) / \sqrt{\varepsilon^2 + |\nabla u_j^{i-1}|^2}(b),$$
$$a_U = \frac{\tau}{h^2} clt(u_j^{i-1})(P) \sqrt{\varepsilon^2 + |\nabla u_j^{i-1}|^2}(P) / \sqrt{\varepsilon^2 + |\nabla u_j^{i-1}|^2}(u),$$
$$a_P = a_W + a_E + a_S + a_N + a_B + a_U + 1, \quad b_P = u_j^{i-1}(P).$$

Remark. By the construction of the system (7.25) the matrix $\mathbf{A}$ is nonsymmetric, but strictly diagonally dominant and thus invertible, so its unique solution always exists. Moreover, the so called L_∞-stability condition is fulfilled for our discrete solution. Namely, let a, b be real constants. If $a \leq \overline{u}_j^0 \leq b$, $j = 0, ..., m$ then $a \leq \overline{u}_j^i \leq b$, $\forall j = 0, ..., m$, $i = 1, 2, ...$ ([17]).

7.5 Discussion on Numerical Experiments

In this section we present and discuss computational results obtained by approximation schemes given in previous sections. First, we are dealing with a phantom-like image sequence consisting of expanding, slightly deforming and moving ellipse with the inner structure in the form of four-petal. We add uniform, impulsive (salt & pepper) and Gaussian noise to frames of the image sequence. The original six-frame sequence and its destroyed version are plotted in first two columns of Figure 7.5. The reconstruction of any noisy frame of the sequence by a usual (still) filtering algorithms (e.g. using comercial software) is a very difficult task and no attempts were successfull. The right column of Figure 7.5 represents the results of nonlinear multiscale analysis (7.14) applied to the noisy sequence after 10 discrete scale steps of our algorithm. A similar result is obtained using space-time filtering equation (7.16).

Next we have applied multiscale analysis models to an in vivo acquired 3D echocardiographic sequence of TomTec Imaging System. In Figures 7.6–7.7 the left ventricular endocardium and the left atrium of one time moment of entire cardiac cycle is visualized. The iso-surfaces corresponding to the interface between cardiac muscle and blood have been computed by the marching cubes method and visualized by a Gouraud shading surface rendering. In the left of Figure 7.6 we plot the echo-volume visualized using the original noisy data, in the middle the result after three discrete scale steps and on the right after nine discrete scale steps of the model (7.14). We have chosen $\tau = 0.2$, $\sigma = 0.0001$ and $h = 1/150$. The next Figure 7.7 is related to the application of the model (7.16) using parameters $\tau = 0.01$, $\varepsilon = 0.0001$ and $h = 1/150$. We plot again original noisy data (left) and the results after three (middle) and six (right) discrete scale steps of our algorithm for the model (7.16).In both cases we look to 5x5 neighborhood of each voxel in order to recognize the Lambertian trajectories of moving points. As one can expect, the resulting shape in Figure 7.7 is little bit more smooth then in Figure 7.6 due to mean curvature flow effect. In [17] the evaluation of accuracy of the proposed method and assumptions of our model from echocardiographic point of view are discussed.

Recently, the 3D + time filtering method has been applied to Real-Time 3D Echo sequences with quite encouraging results. In Figures 7.8 - 7.9 we visualize level surfaces corresponding to un-filtered and filtered left ventricular shapes. We have chosen 5x5 neighbourhood to compute $clt(u)$, $\tau = 0.1$,

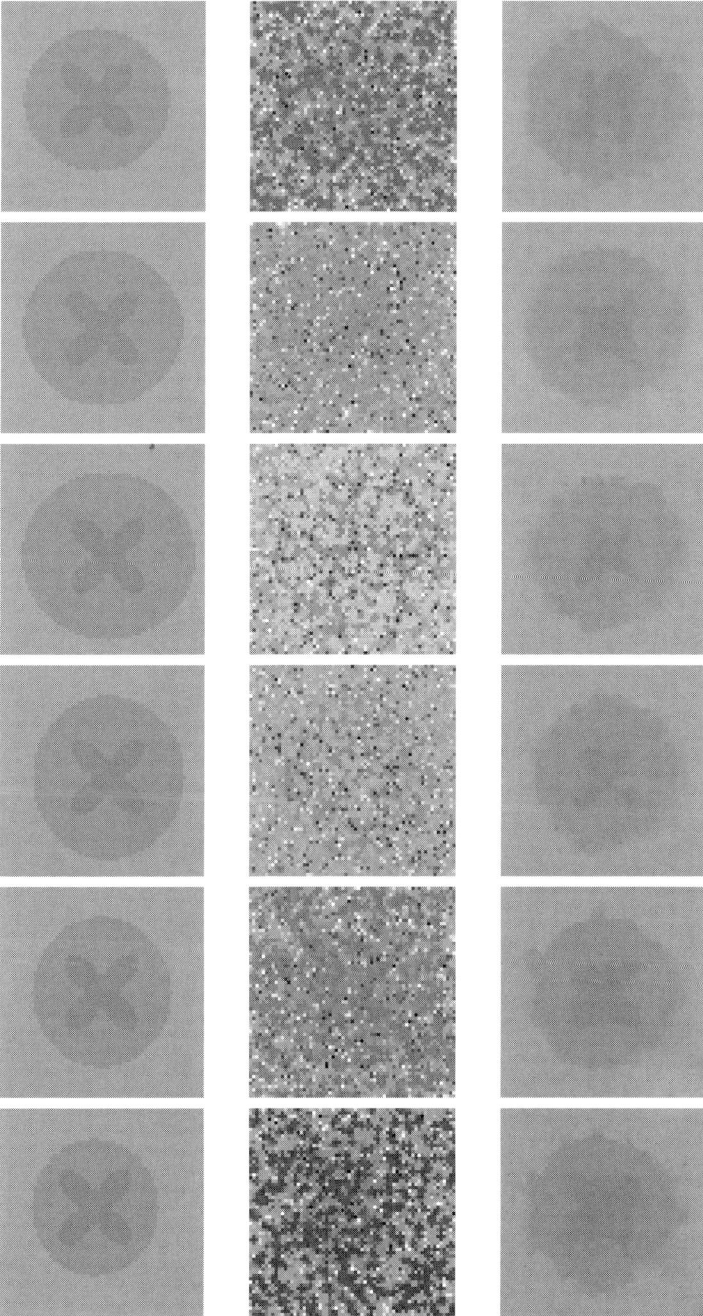

Fig. 7.5. 2D phantom - original (left), noisy (middle) and processed (right) images

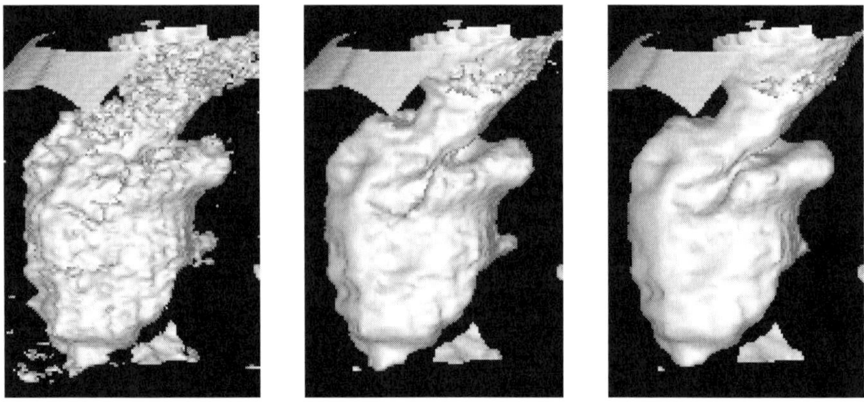

Fig. 7.6. The multiscale analysis of the 7th frame of 3D-echocardiographic image sequence by the equation (7.14)

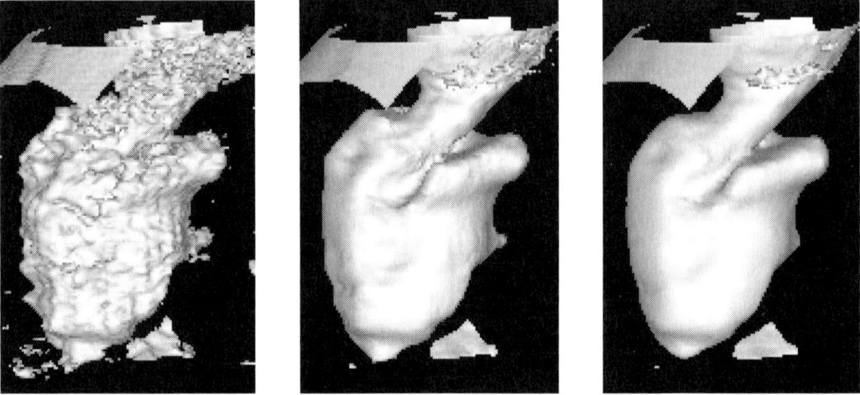

Fig. 7.7. The multiscale analysis of the 7th frame of 3D-echocardiographic image sequence by the equation (7.16)

$\sigma = 0.001$, $h = 1/115$, $K = 2$ and the results are plotted after 3 scale steps of the algorithm for the equation (7.14).

7.6 Preconditioning and Solving of Linear Systems

We finish by a discussion related to solving the linear systems (7.25) which we shortly indicate as

$$\mathbf{A}u = b, \tag{7.27}$$

by means of iterative techniques, focusing our attention on the use of suitable preconditioners. We transform the original system (7.27) into $\mathbf{B}v = c$, where $\mathbf{B} = \mathbf{PAQ}$, $v = \mathbf{Q}^{-1}u$ and $c = \mathbf{P}b$. The matrices $\mathbf{P}$ and $\mathbf{Q}$ are calledd left and right preconditioners, respectively. One preconditioned iteration is

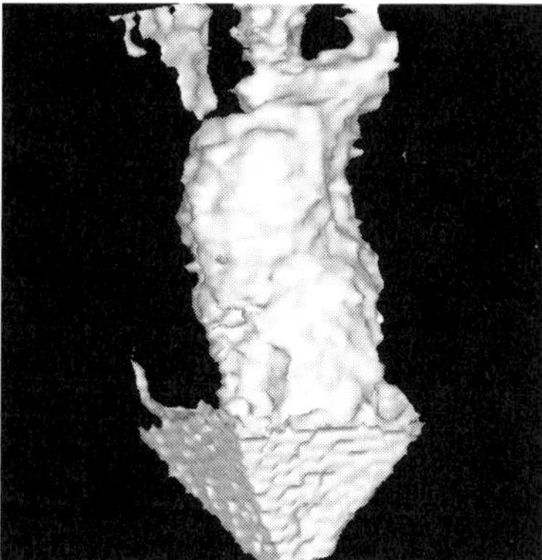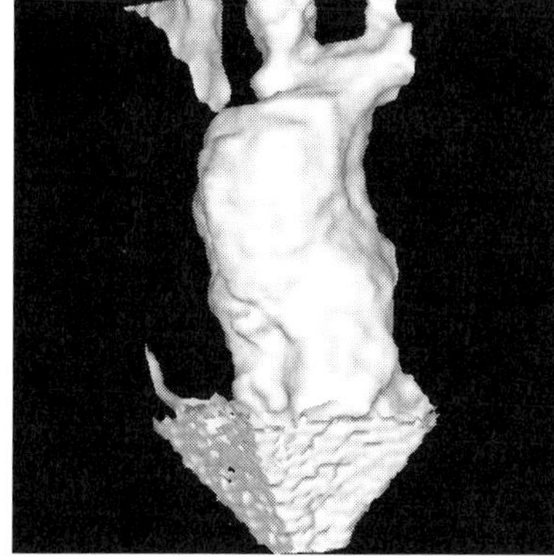

Fig. 7.8. Processing of Real-Time 3D Echo (RT3DE Volumetrics). Visualization of left ventricular surface from 5th cube of the sequence before (left) and after (right) 3D processing by the model (7.14).

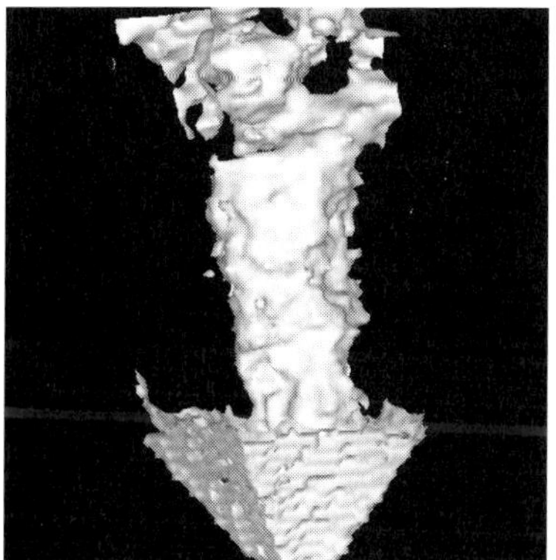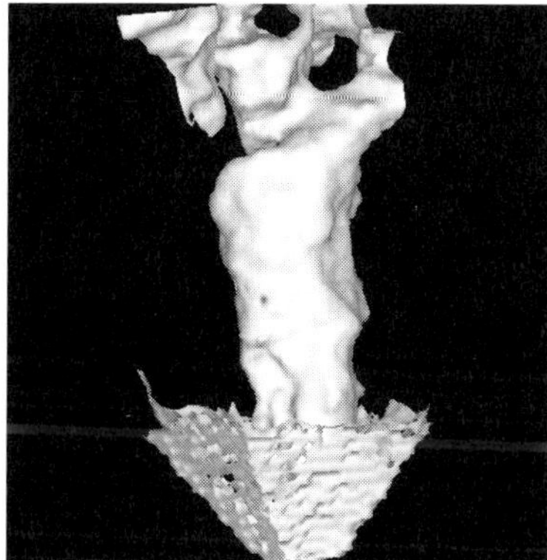

Fig. 7.9. Processing of Real-Time 3D Echo (RT3DE Volumetrics). Visualization of left ventricular surface from 10th cube of the sequence before (left) and after (right) 3D processing by the model (7.14).

usually more expensive than one ordinary iteration. The choice of one particular preconditioner is therefore a trade-off between cost (in time for the trasformations and the preconditionered operations and also in memory) and the effect (in the reduction of number of iterations).

For the 2D image sequences, good performance is achieved also using existing preconditioners. In our comparison we have chosen the classical and most relevant solvers, namely Gauss-Seidel method (GS), conjugate gradient method (CG), biconjugate gradient stabilized method (BICGSTAB), transpose free quasi minimal residual method (TFQMR), generalized minimum residual method (GMRES). At a first investigation we used for each method, when it is possible, the following well-known preconditioners: Right ILU(0) (zero fill-in incomplete LU factorization), Left ILU(0), Right MILU(0) (modified ILU(0)), Left MILU(0) and ILUT(n) (ILU with n-fill in and thresholding). For a detailed discussion on itertive solvers and preconditioners we refer to [16]. In case of GMRES method we allow the restart when the dimension of Krylov subspace is 20. We stop the iterations when the Euclidean norm of the actual residual $r^{(k)} = b - \mathbf{A}u^{(k)}$ satisfies $\|r^{(k)}\| \leq \alpha\|r^{(0)}\|$ with tolerance parameter $\alpha = 0.01$ and $r^{(0)}$ representing the initial residual. We start with $u^{(0)} = 0$. In the 2D testing example (Table 7.1), we process a simple phantom given by a moving noisy circle and for report we choose the time frame from the middle of the sequence. We used $\tau = 0.1$, $\sigma = 0.001$ and $h = 1/128$. In the table, we print the number of matrix-vector product performed until convergence is reached, this number is independent on computer architecture, and the CPU time in seconds (on SUN Sparc 10 workstation) for each complete iterative procedure. We used classical Gauss-Seidel method to compare our preconditioned iterative methods with the widely used direct AOS (Additive Operator Splitting) method ([21]). The AOS method is about three times faster than classical Gauss-Seidel method with the tolerance $\alpha = 0.01$, while from our comparison, it is clear that any preconditioned iterative method is about 10 times faster. In the best case, using the GMRES method we have a speed-up of about 50.

Table 7.1. Comparison of iterative solvers in one scale step of 2D + time algorithm

No.prod/CPU time	GS	CG	BICGSTAB	TFQMR	GMRES
No Precon	265/25.39	94/6.25	98/7.14	204/17.72	114/19.28
Left ILU(0)		20/2.41	20/2.47	18/2.51	17/3.58
Right ILU(0)		No conver	16/2.03	16/2.32	7/1.13
Left ILU(0)		16/1.95	20/2.48	22/3.05	15/3.02
Right MILU(0)		5/0.69	20/2.46	12/1.72	5/0.8
ILUT(5)		–	10/1.57	8/1.11	3/0.51

In 3D case we suggest the following strategy. Approximate inverse $\mathbf{P} \approx \mathbf{A}^{-1}$ is a promising preconditioner for diagonally dominant $\mathbf{A}$ because the entries in $\mathbf{A}^{-1}$ decay rapidly away from diagonal and allows a banded pattern for $\mathbf{P}$. We generate independently the rows of the preconditioner allowing a parallel computation of them. Let p_i denote the column of $\mathbf{P}^{\mathbf{T}}$. Then ideally we would like to have $\mathbf{A}^{\mathbf{T}}p_i = e_i$, where e_i is the i-th column of the identity matrix. From $\mathbf{A}$ we determine some small list of indices I drawn from $\{1, 2, ..., N\}$, where N is equal to the number of unknowns, such that the variables and constraints in I have the most impact on the variable i. Then we solve the small system of equations $\overline{\mathbf{A}^{\mathbf{T}}}\overline{p}_i = \overline{e}_i$, where the bar indicates that we delete all the rows and columns except of those included in I. We let I be i together with all indices of neighbours of node i neglecting those, say j, such that

$$1. |a_{ij} * a_{ji}| \leq thr_1|a_{ii} * a_{jj}|, \quad \text{or} \quad 2. |a_{ij} + a_{ji}| \leq thr_2|a_{ii} + a_{jj}|,$$

where thr_1, thr_2 are user-specified tolerances. The important observation is that the dimension of the small systems does not exceed 7 and so the solution can be computed also in an explicit manner. After the small system is solved, we scatter the entries of the solution $\overline{p_i}$ back to their original coordinate positions in p_i, and we fill in the remaining positions of p_i with zeros. Using compressed sparse row technique for matrices, we have only to store immediately the computed elements and the I indices. As a final observation we may point out that the preconditioner can be computed in a stable manner because the small systems are principal submatrices of $\mathbf{A}$, that is a strictly diagonally dominant M-matrix. For the 3D tests, we stop the iterations by the same criterion as in 2D experimentations and we report the number of matrix-vector products and CPU time in seconds on a SUN Ultra 30. We consider a system arising from the multiscale analysis of ultrasound image sequence with 64^3 voxels in each frame using for the preconditioner $thr_1 = 0.05$ (Table 7.2) and $thr_2 = 0.8$ (Table 7.3). In that cases we observe a good performance of BICGSTAB and GMRES with left preconditioner.

Table 7.2. Comparison of iterative solvers with approximate inverse preconditioner in the processing of one frame of 3D image sequence using the model (7.14)

No.prod/CPU time	BICGSTAB	GMRES
No Precon	145 / 152.27	125 / 274.09
Left	8 / 8.60	9 / 14.63
Right	96 / 76.68	45 / 101.23

Table 7.3. Comparison of iterative solvers with approximate inverse preconditioner in the processing of one frame of 3D image sequence using the model (7.16)

No.Multip/CPU time	BICGSTAB	GMRES
No Precon	145 / 152.27	125 / 274.09
Left	7 / 8.73	7 / 12.58
Right	121 / 118.22	64 / 149.85

Acknowledgment. The authors would like to thank B. Mumm at TomTec for supplying the sequence of 3D Echo data and J. Thomas at Cleveland Clinic Foundation for supplying Real-Time 3D Echo sequences. The work was supported by the Office of Energy Research, Office of Computational and Technology Research, Mathematical, Information and Computational Science Division, Applied Mathematical Sciences Subprogram, of the U.S.

Department of Energy, under Contract No. DE-AC03-76SF00098, by the MI-NOS Project (funded by the European Commission) at CINECA, Bologna, by CNR, Italy, and by the grant VEGA 1/7132/20 in the Slovak Republic.

References

1. Alvarez, L., Guichard, F., Lions, P.L., Morel, J.M.: Axioms and Fundamental Equations of Image Processing. Arch. Rat. Mech. Anal. **123** (1993) 200–257
2. Alvarez, L., Lions, P.L., Morel, J.M.: Image selective smoothing and edge detection by nonlinear diffusion II. SIAM J. Numer. Anal. **29** (1992) 845–866
3. Bänsch, E., Mikula, K.: Adaptivity in 3D image processing. Computing and Visualization in Science (2001)
4. Catté, F., Lions, P.L., Morel, J.M., Coll, T.: Image selective smoothing and edge detection by nonlinear diffusion. SIAM J. Numer. Anal. **29** (1992) 182–193
5. Evans, L.C., Spruck, J.: Motion of level sets by mean curvature I. J. Diff. Geom. **33** (1991) 635–681
6. Guichard, F.: Axiomatisation des analyses multi-échelles d'images et de films. PhD Thesis Univerity Paris IX Dauphine (1994)
7. Handlovičová, A., Mikula, K., Sarti, A.: Numerical solution of parabolic equations related to level set formulation of mean curvature flow. Computing and Visualization in Science **1**, No. 2 (1999) 179–182
8. Handlovičová, A., Mikula, K., Sgallari, F.: Variational numerical methods for solving nonlinear diffusion equations arising in image processing, Journal of Visual Communication and Image Representation (2001)
9. Kačur, J., Mikula, K.: Solution of nonlinear diffusion appearing in image smoothing and edge detection. Applied Numerical Mathematics **17** (1995) 47–59
10. Kichenassamy, R.: The Perona-Malik paradox. SIAM J. Appl. Math. **57**, No.5 (1997) 1328–1342
11. Malladi, R., Sethian, J.A., Vemuri, B.: Shape modeling with front propagation: a level set approach. IEEE Trans. Pattern Analysis Machine Intelligence **17**, No.2 (1995) 158–174
12. Mikula, K., Ramarosy, N.: Semi-implicit finite volume scheme for solving nonlinear diffusion equations in image processing. Numerische Mathematik (2001)
13. Mikula, K., Sarti, A., Lamberti, C.: Geometrical diffusion in 3D-echocardiography. Proceedings of ALGORITMY'97 - Conference on Sci. Comp., Zuberec, Slovakia (1997) 167–181
14. Perona, P., Malik, J., Scale space and edge detection using anisotropic diffusion. In Proc. IEEE Computer Society Workshop on Computer Vision (1987)
15. Rudin, L.I., Osher, S., Fatemi, E.: Nonlinear total variation based noise removal algorithms. Physica D **60** (1992) 259–268
16. Saad, Y.: Iterative methods for sparse linear systems. PWS Publ. Comp. (1996)
17. Sarti, A., Mikula, K., Sgallari, F.: Nonlinear multiscale analysis of 3D echocardiographic sequences. IEEE Transactions on Medical Imaging **18**, No. 6 (1999) 453–466
18. Sarti,A., Ortiz de Solorzano,C., Lockett, S. and Malladi, R.: A Geometric Model for 3-D Confocal Image Analysis. IEEE Transactions on Biomedical Engineering **45**, No. 12, (2000), 1600–1610

19. Sarti,A., Malladi,R., Sethian,J.A.: Subjective Surfaces: A Method for Completing Missing Boundaries. Proceedings of the National Academy of Sciences of the United States of America,Vol 12, N.97, pag. 6258-6263, 2000.
20. Sethian, J.A.: Level Set Methods and Fast Marching Methods. Evolving Interfaces in Computational Geometry, Fluid Mechanics, Computer Vision, and Material Science. Cambridge University Press (1999)
21. Weickert, J., Romeny, B.M.t.H., Viergever, M.A.: Efficient and reliable schemes for nonlinear diffusion filtering. IEEE Trans. on Image Processing **7** (1998)

Appendix

Color Plates

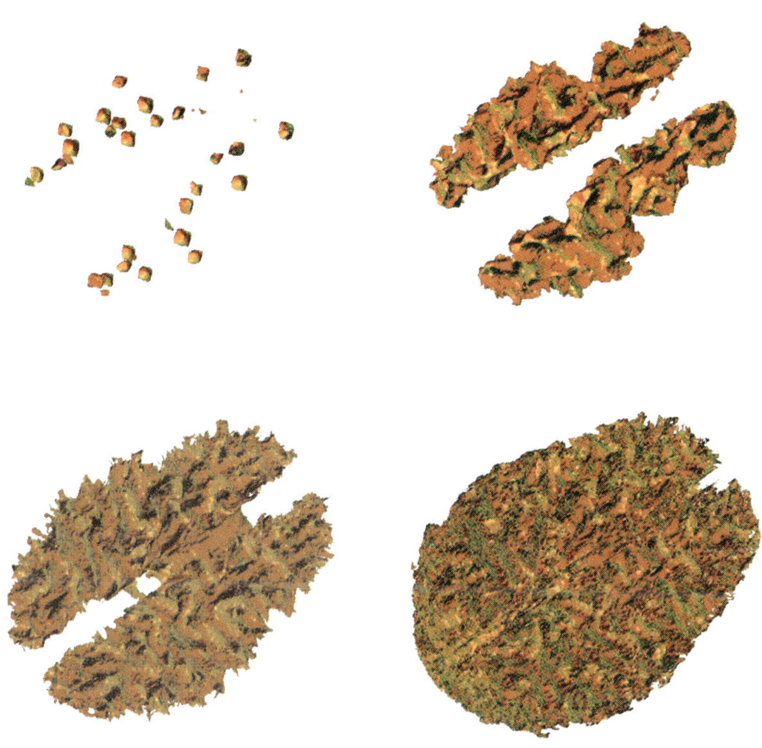

Plate 1. Evolutionary sequence showing the brain reconstruction. Here we have rendered particular level sets of the function $T(x, y, z)$; the surfaces in the left-to-right top-to-bottom order correspond to the values $T(x, y, z) = 0.01, 0.125, 0.25, 0.75$. (*R. Malladi and J.A. Sethian, p. 8.*)

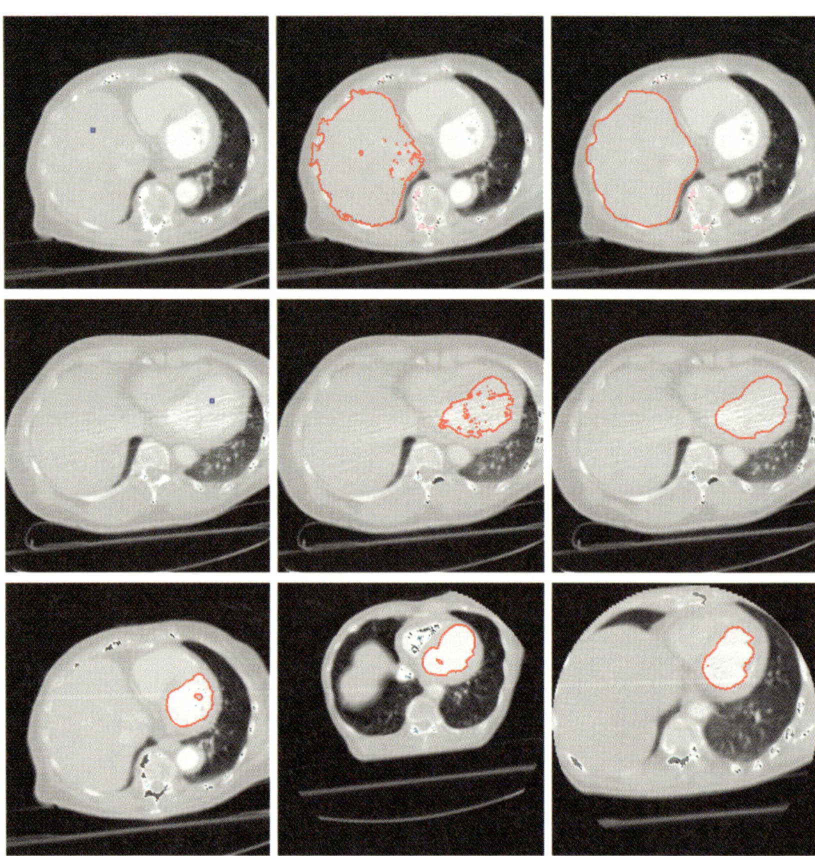

Plate 2. *2D* examples of our two-stage shape recovery scheme. From left-to-right in the first two rows we show (a) the initial mouse click, (b) the end of Stage # 1, and (c) the end of Stage #2. In the last row we show three more converged results. (*R. Malladi and J.A. Sethian, p. 11.*)

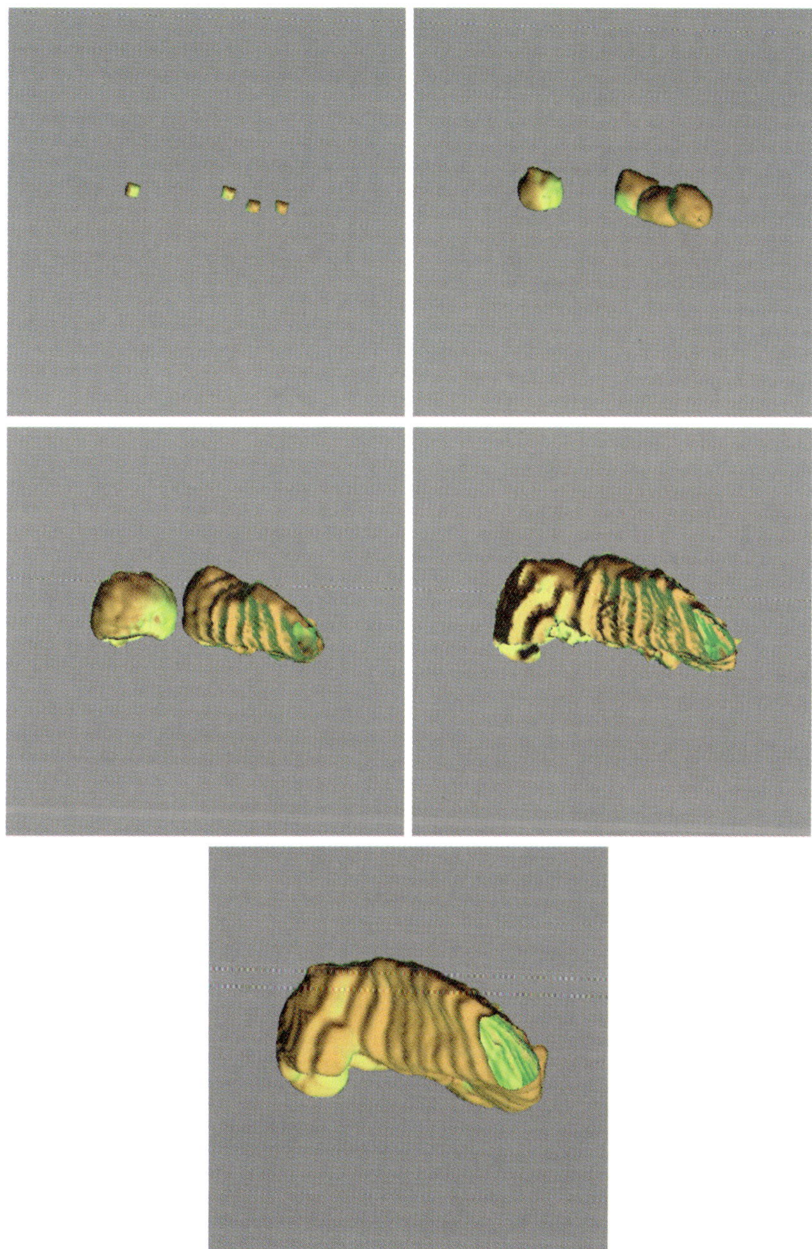

Plate 3. The two-stage shape recovery in $3D$: the first four surfaces are the level sets $\{T(x, y, z) = 0.01\}$, 0.035, 0.07, and 0.10 respectively. This also marks the end of Stage #1. The result of solving the level set shape recovery equation for a few steps is shown in the final figure (*R. Malladi and J.A. Sethian, p. 14.*)

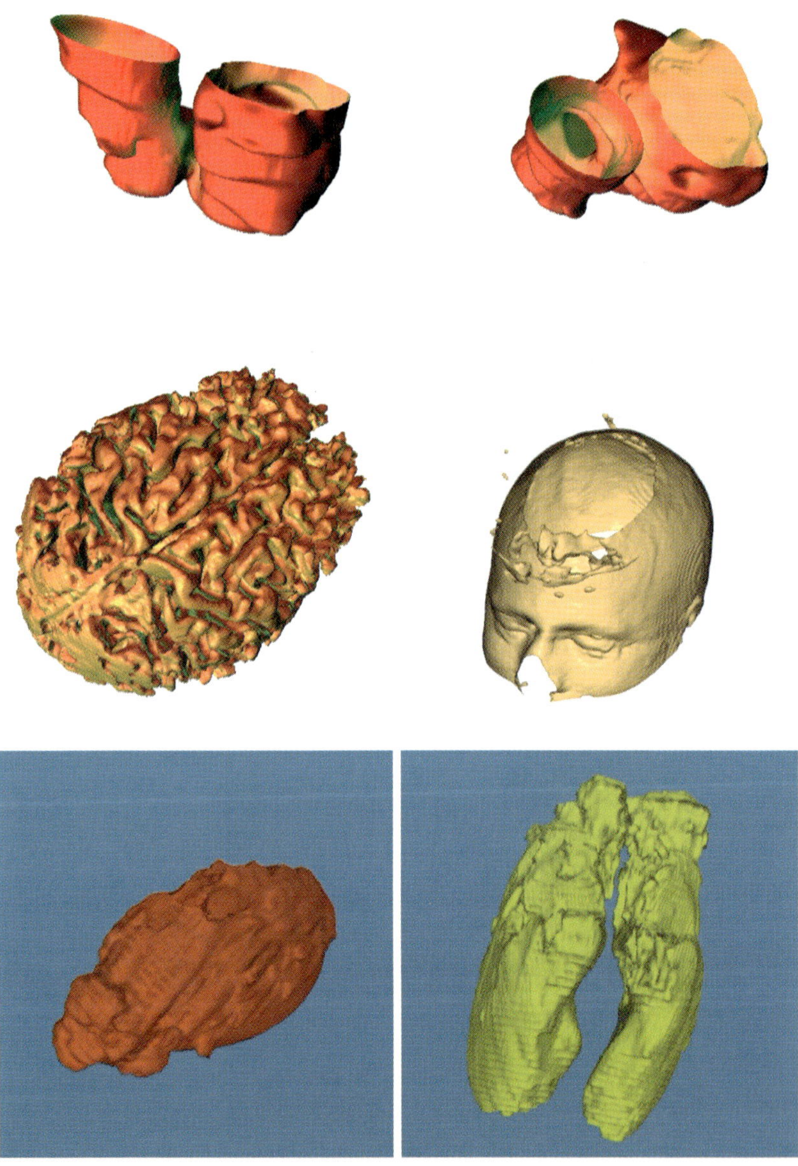

Plate 4. More examples of 3D shape recovery. (*R. Malladi and J.A. Sethian, p. 16.*)

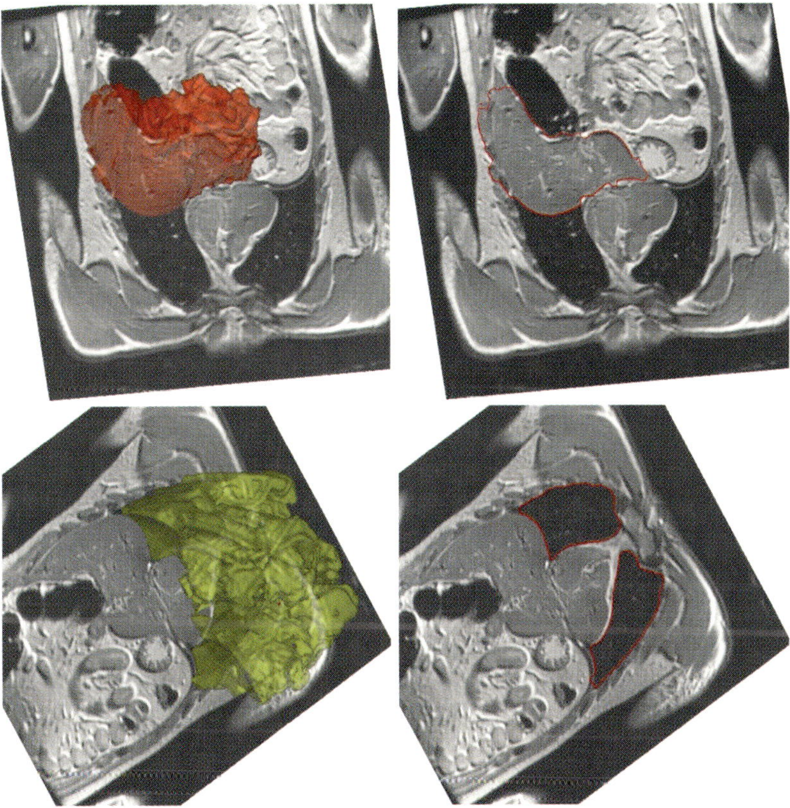

Plate 5. $3D$ results superimposed on a particular $2D$ image slice. (*R. Malladi and J.A. Sethian, p. 17.*)

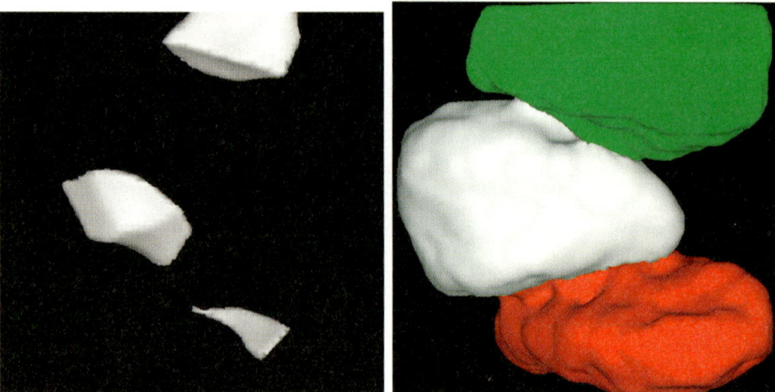

Plate 6. The refined clusters after processing with the multiple interface flow. (a)Left: three distinct shapes after the *erode* operation. (b)Right: three different cells have been recognized and segmented. (*Ortiz de Solorzano, Malladi, and Lockett, p. 30.*)

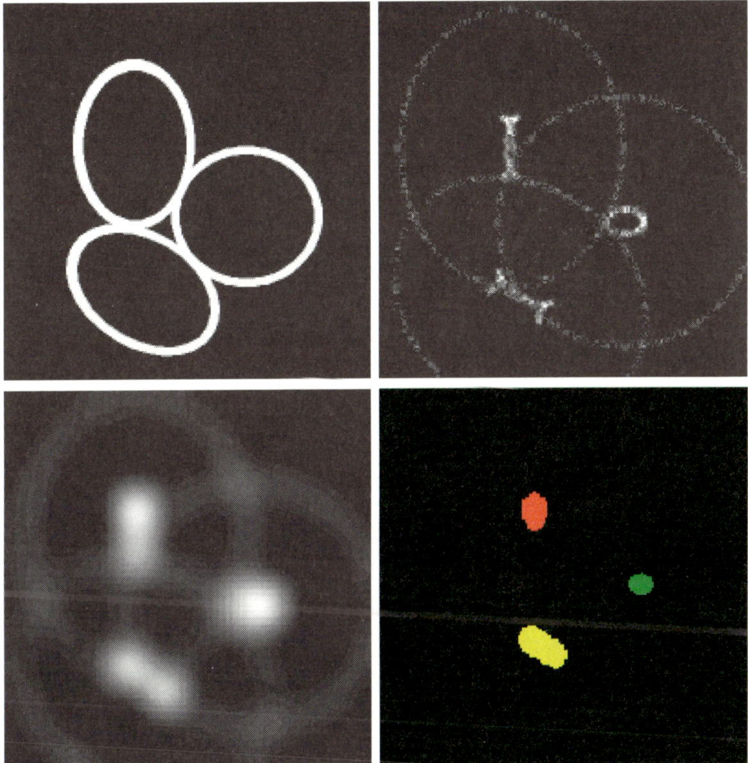

Plate 7. Nuclear segmentation using a computer generated image. (a)Top left: simulation of a cluster of three surface stained nuclei. (b) Top right: Hough Transform of (a), where gradients in the original image are projected using and estimate of the object size. (c) Bottom left: Gaussian filtered version of (b). (d) Bottom Left: Final seeds obtained using a morphological peak detection algorithm. (*Ortiz de Solorzano, Malladi, and Lockett, p. 35.*)

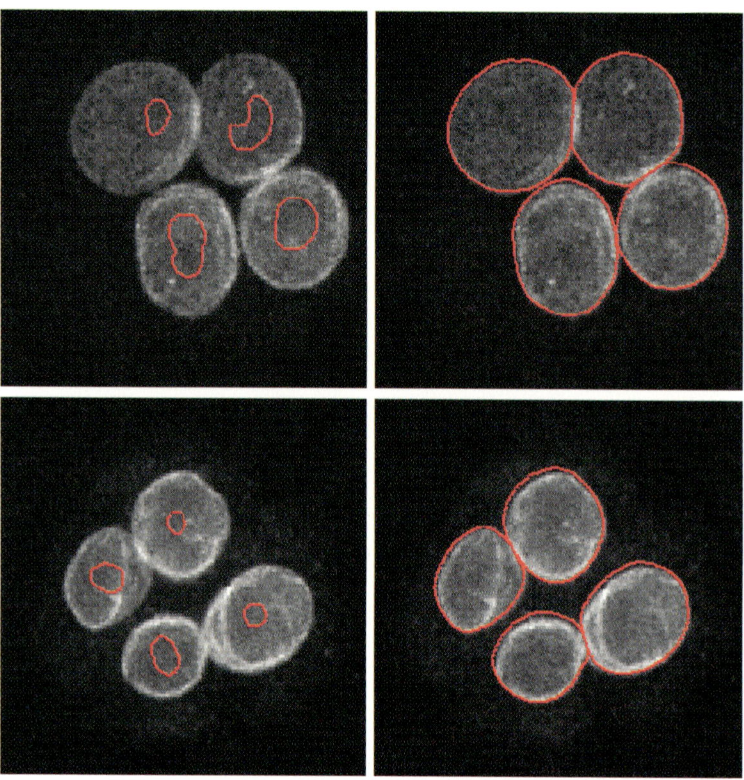

Plate 8. Examples of the segmentation results on real images from cultured lamin stained cells. (a)and (c) Left column: Original images with the automatically detected seeds. (b) and (d)Right column: Results, overimposed on the original images. (*Ortiz de Solorzano, Malladi, and Lockett, p. 38.*)

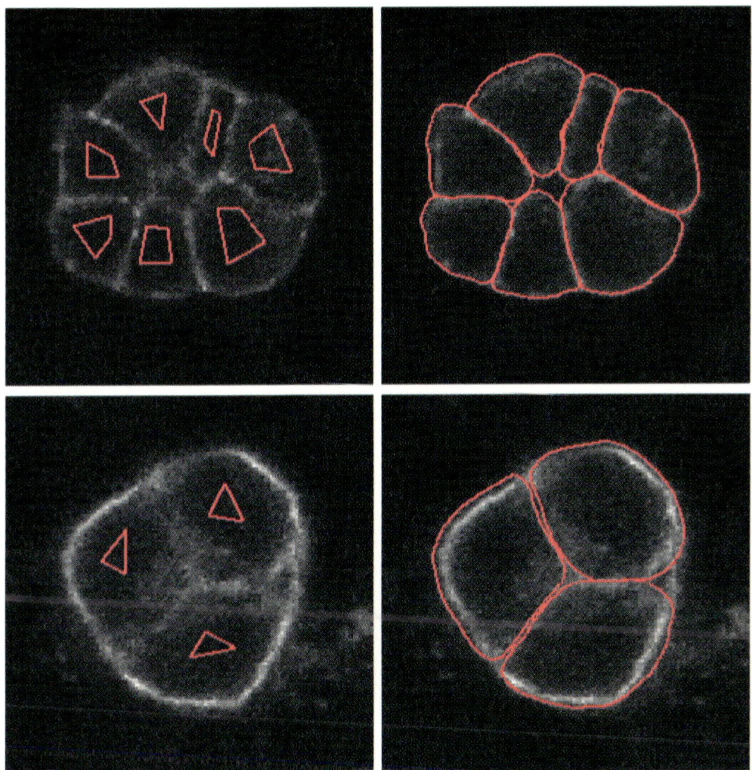

Plate 9. Examples of the segmentation results on cultured aGb1 integrin stained cells. (a) and (c) Left column: Original images with the interactively detected seeds. (b) and (d) Right column: Results, overimposed on the original images. The white arrows in figure (b) show concavities that were followed by the algorithm. (*Ortiz de Solorzano, Malladi, and Lockett, p. 39.*)

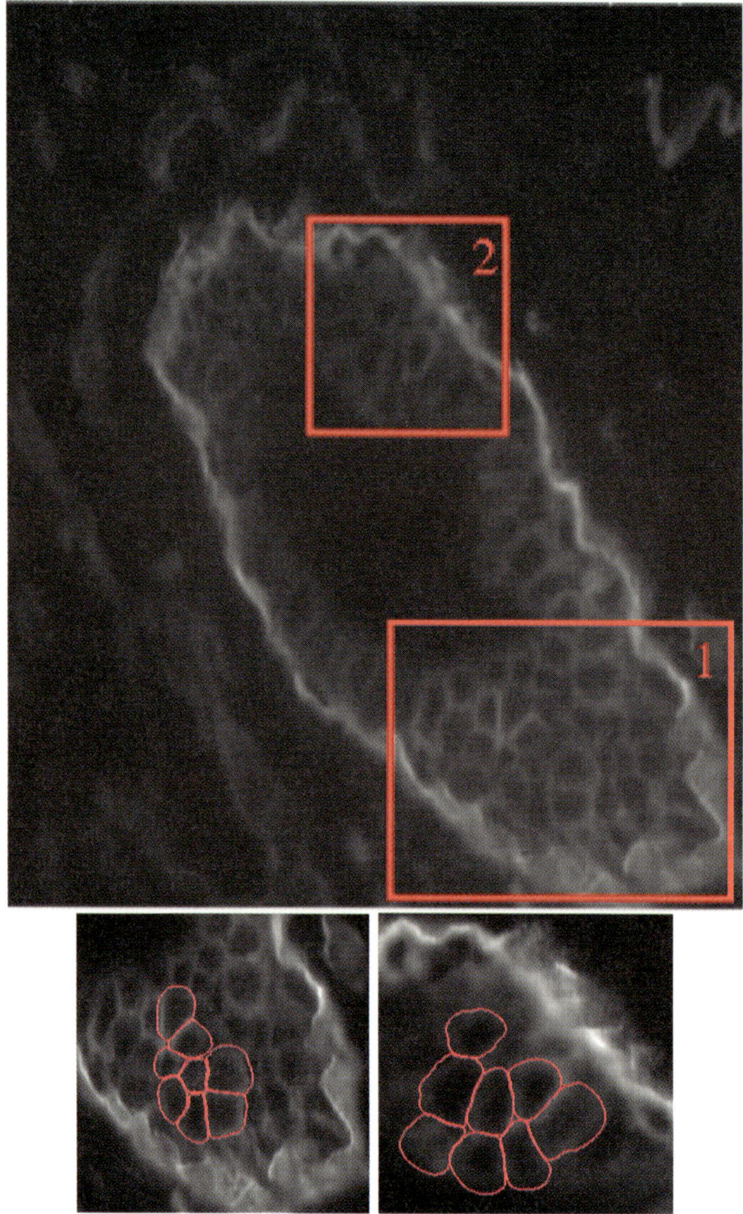

Plate 10. Example of the segmentation results on two parts (b) and (c) of a mouse mammary tissue stained for a6b1 integrin. (a) Top: Original image. (b) and (c) Bottom: show Results on interactively seeded nuclei from two parts of image a. (*Ortiz de Solorzano, Malladi, and Lockett, p. 42.*)

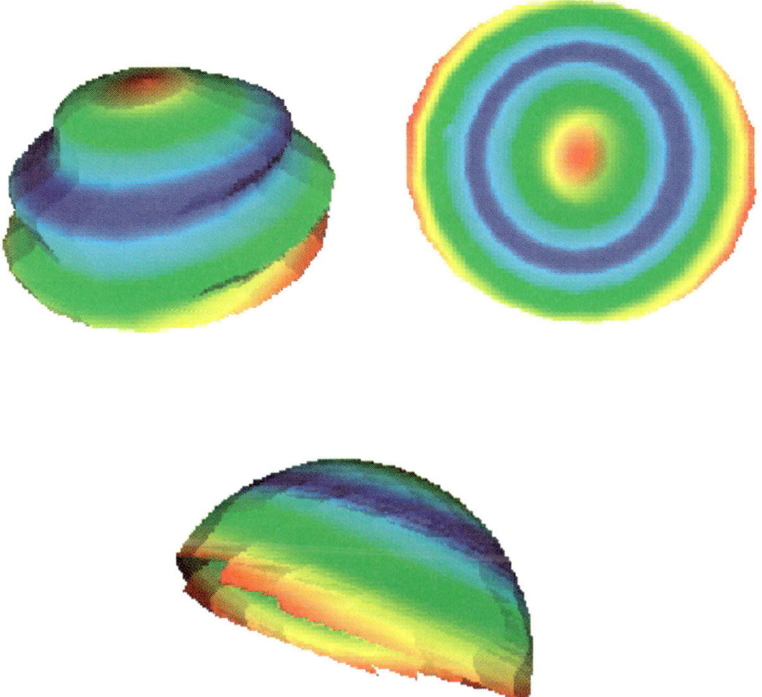

Plate 11. Comparison between different flattening approaches. **Top left:** Original sphere-like surface. **Top right:** Planar flattening with matching error (Stress) = 0.0132. **Bottom:** Mapping onto a sphere with matching error (Stress) = 0.00945. (*Elad and Kimmel, p. 79.*)

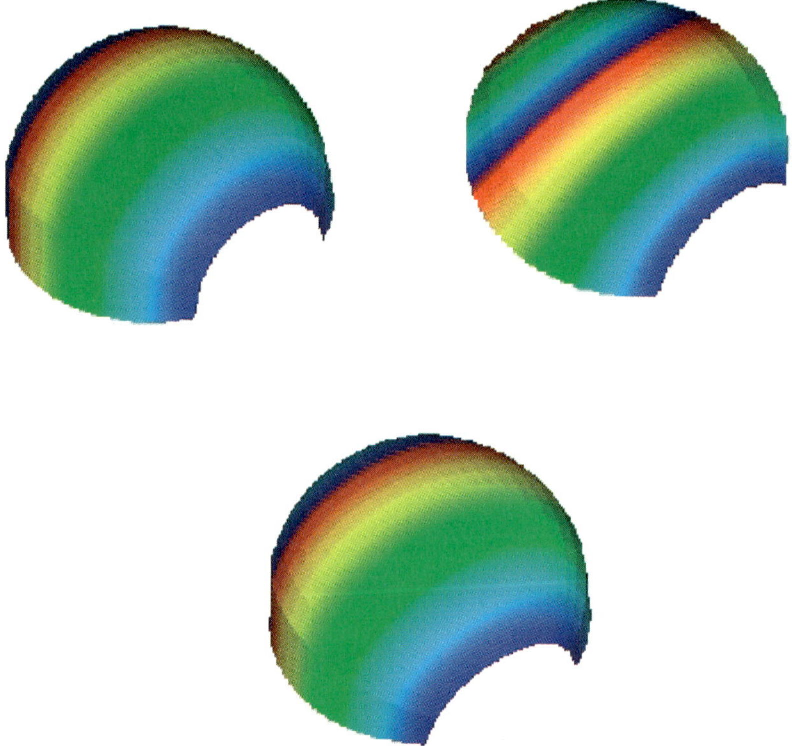

Plate 12. Sphere flattening using Euclidean and arc-length distances. **Top left:** Original surface. **Top right:** Cox [3] approach using Euclidean distance. **Bottom:** Our approach using the arc-length geodesic distance on the target sphere. (*Elad and Kimmel, p. 83.*)

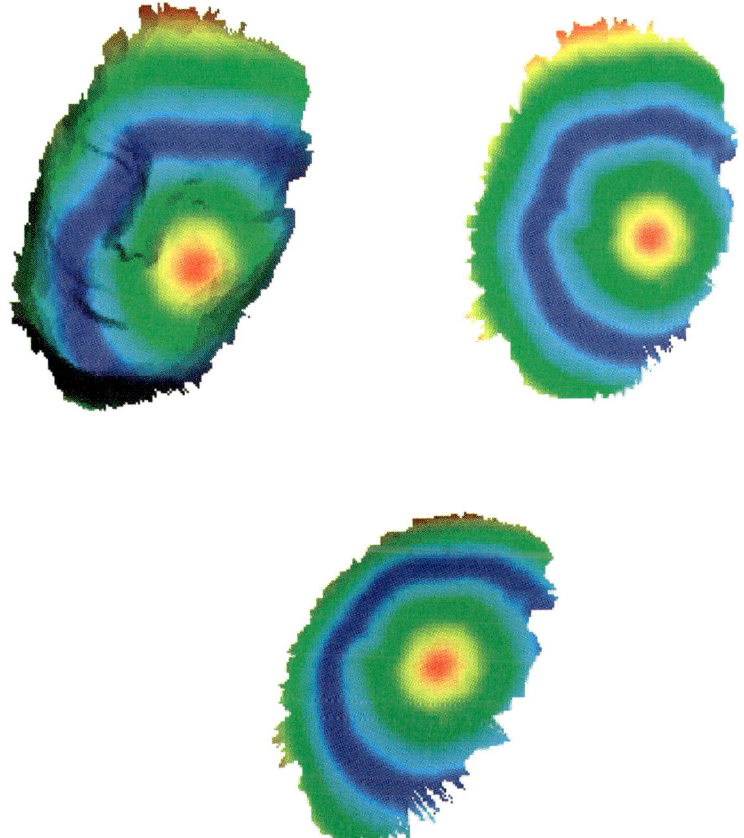

Plate 13. Comparison between different flattening approaches for a human face. **Top left:** Original surface. **Top right:** Planar flattening (Stress = 0.000314). **Bottom:** mapping onto a sphere (Stress = 0.000312). (*Elad and Kimmel, p. 85.*)

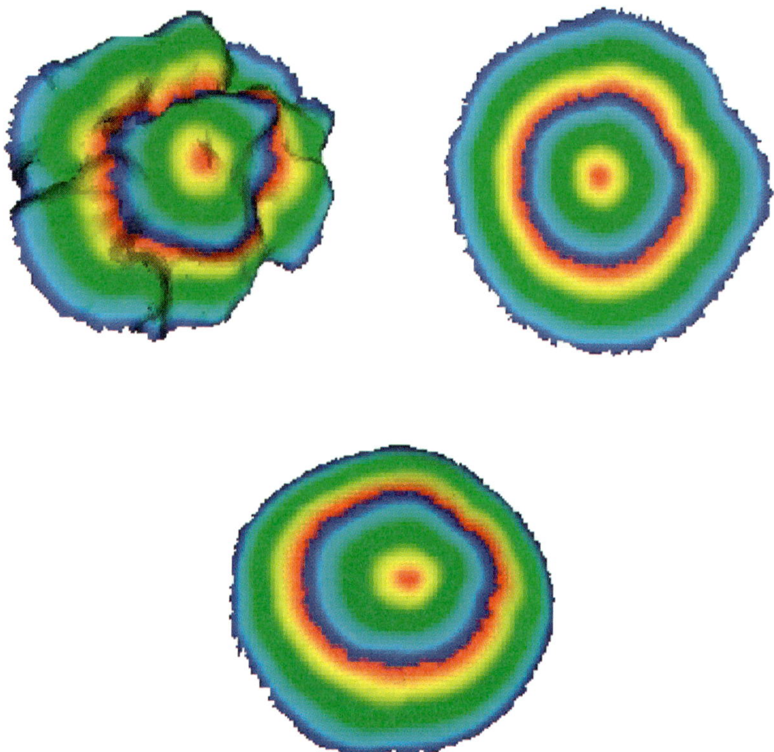

Plate 14. Flattening a section of a human cortex. **Top left:** Original surface (3000 vertices). **Top right:** Planar flattening (Stress = 0.0020). **Bottom:** Mapping onto a sphere (Stress = 0.0011). (*Elad and Kimmel, p. 87.*)

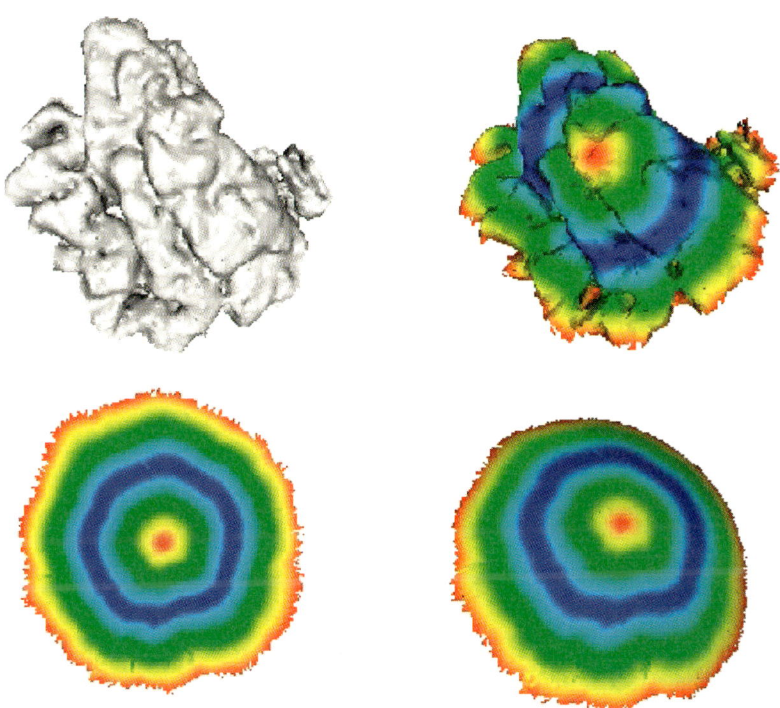

Plate 15. Flattening a section of a human cortex. **Top left:** Original surface (20000 vertices). **Top right:** Decimated surface (5000 vertices). **Bottom left:** Planar flattening (Stress = 0.0038). **Bottom right:** Mapping onto a sphere (Stress = 0.0022). (*Elad and Kimmel, p. 88.*)

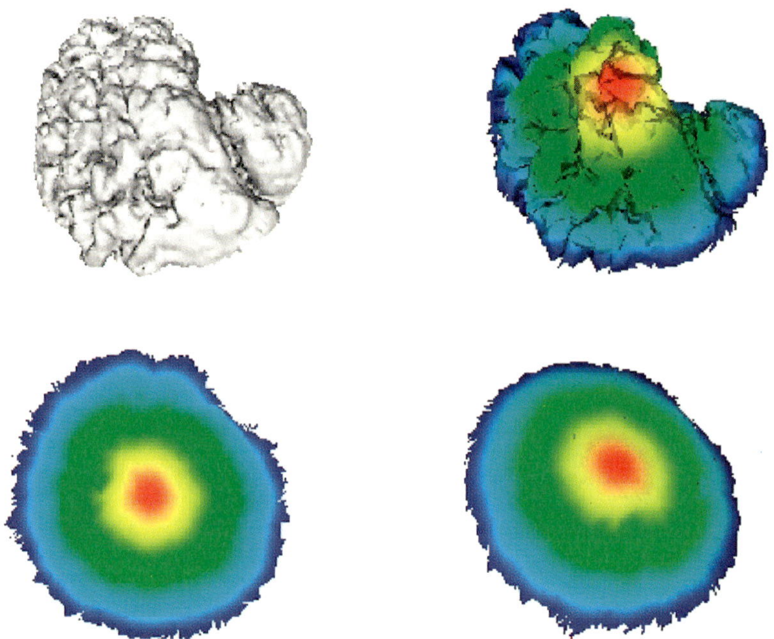

Plate 16. Flattening a section of a human cortex. **Top left:** Original surface (56000 vertices). **Top right:** Decimated surface (3500 vertices). **Bottom left:**Planar flattening (Stress = 0.0088). **Bottom right:** Mapping onto a sphere (Stress = 0.0060). (*Elad and Kimmel, p. 89.*)

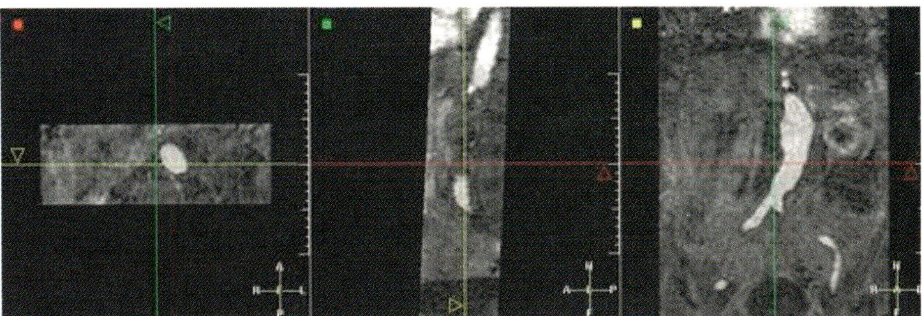

Plate 17. Three orthogonal slices of the aorta MR dataset. (*Deschamps and Cohen, p. 105.*)

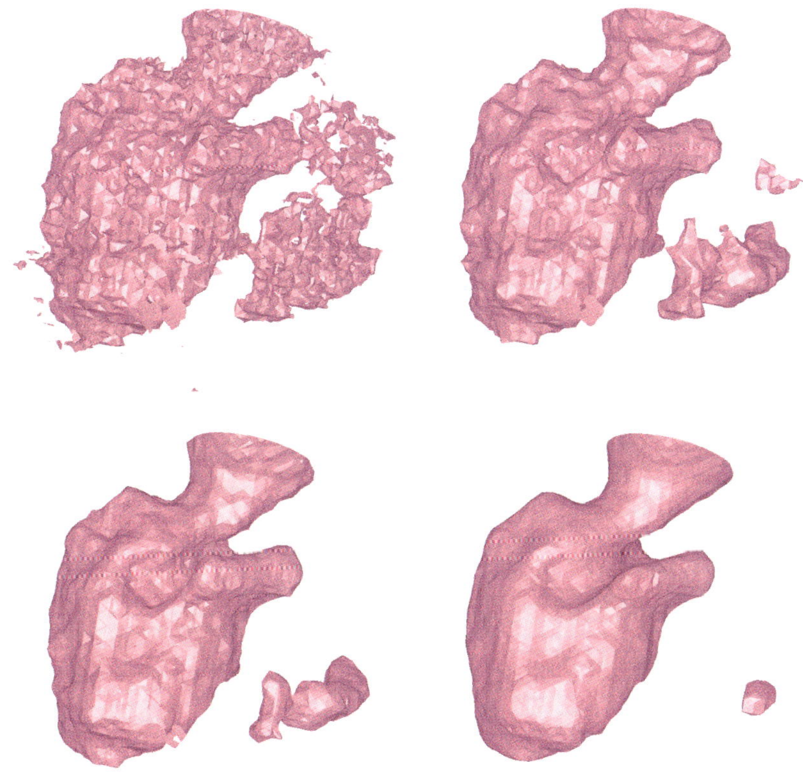

Plate 18. Smoothing of the human left ventricle by anisotropic diffusion. We visualize correponding level surfaces in 0th, 2nd, 4th and 8th discrete steps of semi-implicit finite element algorithm ([3]). (*Sarti, Mikula, Sgallari, and Lamberti, p. 112.*)

Druck: Strauss Offsetdruck, Mörlenbach
Verarbeitung: Schäffer, Grünstadt